Money, Gifts & Sex

A Sugar Daddy & Sugar Baby in a
New Dress Among the African Australians

SATURNINO ONYALA

Money, Gifts And Sex: A Sugar Daddy And Sugar Baby
In A New Dress Among African Australians
Saturnino Onyala

978-0-6484367-3-7 (PBK)
978-0-6484367-4-4 (HBK)

First published in April 2020

April 2020
Melbourne, Australia

Printed and bound by IngramSpark Australia

About The Author

Saturnino is a South Sudanese Australian who came to Australia as a refugee in 2003. By obtaining a Master degree in Social Science, specializing in International Development from RMIT University Melbourne, the author was exposed to global cultural trends. This in turn, inspired him to create conversations around hidden and undocumented aspects of African cultures and historical milestones. His first book *The History and Expressive Cultures of the Acholi of South Sudan* was a reflection of valuable knowledge gained through a number of research and conversations with elders in the community. His second book *A Short Social and Cultural Anthropology of the Northern Luo of South Sudan* explored the cultural frameworks of South Sudanese Lou people and their untold stories.

About The Author

Abstract

This book systematically documents the practices of African males and females, who are currently involved in the practice of "sugar daddy" and "sugar baby" in Australia under the new names: "brother or uncle" and "sister". The communal talk about sugar daddies and sugar babies among African Australians, has prompted me to do research and write this book. I believe that my findings will be useful and applicable to other Africans living in America, Canada and Europe, if they are also involved in the same practices. This book will examine their occurrence, acceptability, as well as the perceived reasons behind the practices.

The research covered 80 participants from diverse African groups, from both sexes, living in Australia. Formerly, I planned to interview 200 Africans but due to communication barriers, sensitivity of the topic, lack of intimacy between researcher and participants and distances between researcher and informants, I was then forced to reduce the number from 200 to 80 participants. The other reason for reducing the number of participants was that I expected I may not get correct answers to the questions from some women. And this has been revealed during my interviews with the people; I have experienced difficulties getting the complete facts about current practices of sugar daddies and sugar babies among Africans living in Australia.

Data on the participants' views, opinions and experiences of being a sugar daddy or sugar baby was collected using individual face-to-face interviews and by telephone. I have avoided using emails as a means of data collection for fear of exposing personal details and breaking confidentiality.

When the collection of data was completed, the researcher (Onyala) then analysed it; the research revealed that although some men and women practise as "sugar daddies" and "sugar babies", the African women in Australia do not practise as "sugar mummies". The research found that not all the African men and women in Australia practise "sugar daddy" and "sugar baby", but some of them do — the majority are single mothers and some married men, as well as some married women. I used to hear and read that in Africa there are "sugar mummies" too, so this finding made me ask myself, why are there no African sugar mummies in Australia? The common answer that I got was that African women in Australia do not have enough annual income that would qualify them to be "sugar mummies".

It is assumed that for an African woman to become a sugar mummy and to be considered rich, her annual income must be between AUD$150,000 to $300,000. Statistics suggest that the annual income for African women living in Australia ranges between AUD$50,000 to $100,000. Therefore, this means whatever annual income African women receive from their standard jobs it is not enough to become a sugar mummy.

Interestingly, the research shows that African girls aged 18-26, who live in Australia do not practise the work of a sugar baby; they depend on Centrelink income and wages from their jobs. In contrast, research shows that some African females aged 27-65 do practise sugar baby — these include some of the housewives as mentioned above.

More importantly, study shows that most of the income African sugar babies receive from their sugar daddies is used for beautification of their body and house. The remaining balance is used for rent, bills, medication, food, school uniforms and mortgages (where applicable). Having said this, I would like to point out that African women in Australia are not as rich as the Anglo-Australian sugar mummies, which would allow them to attract and flirt with males.

It appears that the perceived reasons and acceptability of sugar babies by some African women are many, but the most common ones consist of the following: survival, financial difficulty, finding additional money to send to relatives overseas, rent, bills, material wants, sexual fulfilments, reduction of stress, separation from partner, love and so on.

However, the primary objective of this book is to provide a broad overview of African sugar daddies and African sugar babies' practices here in Australia. It is hoped that the book would be used to provide a framework to prevent escalation of sugar daddy and sugar baby practices among the African Australians –who call Australia their new home.

Given the increase of sugar daddies and sugar babies among African Australians, which may have significant implications in the potential killing by ex-husbands of sugar babies, it is necessary for African males and females, as well as service providers, to understand the underlying perceptions and consequences/impacts that such practices could bring on African communities. And this is one of the reasons for writing this informative book.

Therefore, the writer thinks that it is better to develop culturally and socially acceptable intervention programmes at Local Government and State or Territory levels, before these practices spread among the community. One could ask, "How would this be possible, since sugar daddy and sugar baby practices are accepted by the Australia people?" It is true that to the Australians, there is nothing unlawful with sugar daddy and sugar baby practices, but we could still help our African Australians understand better. It is assumed that if culturally and socially acceptable programmes are developed, current and future African generations would be rescued from such bad practices. The question would be then, "What percentage of Africans males and females would be rescued?" This question may need further research.

Acknowledgement

I started writing this book in May 2019 as a result of a "hot" topic being discussed underground by the African Australians. However, there have been no open discussions, since the topic is humiliating to the communities.

First and foremost, I would like to acknowledge the African men and women who have contributed to the success of this book through phone conversations and by responding to text messages. I personally appreciated the level of disclosure that was given about unspoken relationships, which resulted in the publication of this unique, informative and educational book.

However, I want to inform the readers that the names of men and women who have contributed are held in strict confidence for the simple reason that the topic discussed is too sensitive for the African community in Australia. It is done this way to avoid some members of community pointing a finger at contributors.

It was a privilege for me to have the chance to put pen to paper and raise an unheard voice about sugar daddy and sugar baby practices, which are in full swing among African Australians. I thank those who disclosed to me how a sugar daddy and a sugar baby attract each other, the level of secrecy and how the practices have grown, despite the challenges they face and continue to face. I feel particularly grateful to all informants who have contributed to the completion of this book. Without them I would have not reached where I have reached today.

I would like to register my profound gratitude and appreciation to Mr Luke Harris, a graphic designer from Working Type Studio in Eltham, Melbourne

(Australia), for his support and guidance. I welcomed his positive and insightful suggestions on how to improve the book. I first met Luke Harris when I was in the process of designing and laying out my first book entitled *The History and Expressive Cultures of the Acholi of South Sudan*.

It is commonly said that every success in life has challenges; I was not an exception. One of the greatest challenges I faced in my research about this sensitive topic was gaining access to all Africans who are currently living in Australia. Although there were communication restrictions here and there, nevertheless, several people finally made it possible for me to share their inner feelings and ideas, opinions, perceptions and the rich knowledge they have about African sugar daddy and sugar baby practices back home in Africa, as well as in Australia

Lest I forget, I also want to thank my family members for their patience by not disturbing me in my research and when compiling the data. However, it was fortunate that my family members did not know the subject matter of my research because if they were to know, they would have negative reactions about it. So I was very careful in handling the articles and books I was reading that were covering the subject matter of this topic. I then took advantage of their ignorance, which made it possible for me to write without fear. I am pretty sure that if they were to know that I was writing a book about sugar daddy and sugar baby practices, they would have 'hit my head with a mahogany stick' and burnt all the research papers. They would do this because in many African cultures, no one can discuss or write about sugar relationships in the family home. Many Africans believe that the work of a sugar daddy and sugar baby is bad for individuals as well as for the community, because it often ends up in the death (killing) of one party (and women are usually the victims), or death of both. This can highlight the complexities and outright risks with these relationships where one party gives money or property to the other person in exchange for sex.

I would also like to thank the Australian Government for passing the law of forbidding family violence —because hitting a head of someone with a mahogany stick would be considered as family violence. I believe this is one of the factors that protected me, otherwise my family members might have taken the law into their own hands, should they know the subject matter of my book. Therefore the research and data collection about African sugar daddies and sugar babies has challenged me both intellectually and personally.

Finally, I am grateful to my late mother, Laura Akwero Onek, who passed away in Melbourne, Australia, on 23ʳd June 2019, at the age of 91. During her lifetime in Australia, she managed to save some money in her bank account. So, after her death and funeral expenses, I was able to use her funds through her Will for the publication of this book. My mother was a true mother and a person who had sincere love and care in her heart for her children and grand-children. I therefore dedicate this book to her memory.

Table of Contents

Saturnino Onyala, the Man
"Autobiographical sketch"

I was born on the 01/01/1951 in Licari-Obbo. Licari is situated on a plateau. People settled here because the soil is very fertile. Secondly, there is a good number of games which provide meat for the inhabitants—food staff in Laciri is adequate. There are no schools in Licari. All children study in a 'Bush school' in Oyere, which is about four to five miles from Licari. My father was a great hunter and farmer. He also worked in coffee farm at Obbo between 1960 and 1962. Later, he went to work as a game ranger in Kasese-Uganda.

I started Primary One in a bush school in 1960 when I was already ten years old. Joining school was a problem to me because teachers said I was above the age of starting school. Fortunately, the God of my father had "lain stomach up". A police officer, Lazario the brother of Adik-Diko-moi, of Licari, who headed the police who were keeping peace at the time of enrolling school pupil told the teachers to register me in Primary One. With the authority of Lazario, I was enrolled in Primary One. Although my father was working in coffee farm at Obbo, we did not have a bicycle. So I always walked to school. Sometimes I met elephants and buffaloes on my way to school. My 'Bush school' teachers were Opeko of Obbo, and Teodoro Lo-um, (he was often called by his nickname, Otyien) of Pajok. As the Acholi said, it is the children from poor families are the ones who are brighter in class. Truly, I was a bright child and all my teachers liked me.

In 1963, I passed the examinations which were for the pupils of Palwar, Pajok, Obbo, Magwi, Omeo and Panyikwara. At that time, Acholi children from different families completed their primary two from village schools, after which they did the examinations to join Palotaka Elementary School. From every bush school, teachers chose forty five Primary Two pupils who scored high marks to join Palotaka Elementary School. I studied in Palotaka Elementary School for six months. Later, government transferred one teacher from Juba to Palotaka. This teacher had two boys who were in Primary Three. That year, Mr. Labuk was the headmaster of Palotaka Elementary School. Shortly, the new teacher asked the headmaster to remove two pupils from Primary Three so that there was space for his boys in the class. I do not know how the headmaster's eyes functioned! His sight fell on me and one of my friends, Michael Oyuru of Pajok Paitenge. The headmaster called both of us in his office and informed us that each of us should go back to study in the village schools. Michael Oyuru went back to study in Pajok village school while I went to Oyere village school.

The Mwony Anya-nya rebel had started in 1962. In 1964, my mother, Laura Onek, fled with my two sisters and I to Palabek Akeli-kongo in Uganda. Refugee life was not easy. A short while later, the Palabek people started calling us *Agono ki Lokung* (I came via Lukung). In 1964, I resumed Primary Three in Palabek Kal Primary School. All the same, life was hard because the wife of my Uncle, Dr Mario Tokwaro, with whom I lived, used to deny me breakfast every morning. She did not want me to wash my face with the water in her pot. At the same time, I was also a mass boy at Palabek Mission. When it was time for me to go to school or church, I washed my face from a bore hole, or with dew using cassava leaves. In 1965 I went to study in Palabek Padwat where I lived with my mother's sister called Mrs. Imerigiana Lalaa. When I realised that I may not have a good place to study from, I joined *Pakele Minor Seminary* in 1966 when Father Leopoldo Anywar of Amika Magwi was the Rector of Pakele Minor Seminary. When Father Father Leopoldo identified me as a bright boy, he appointed me as a storekeeper of student's food store. Later, Father Hillary Loswat Oboma of Lokoro, realised that the Parish Priest of Pakele Mission wanted to remove me out of the seminary because I gave food to students whom he wanted to punish by starvation. It is true that when the Parish Priest ordered that there was no food for students the following day, I gave much food staff to be prepared for their meals because I thought that if they eat much today, they would not feel very hungry the following day. In 1967 Father Hillary Loswat Oboma, transferred me to *Nadiket Minor Seminary* in Moroto, where I completed Primary seven. In 1969, I went to study in *Lacor Senior Seminary* Gulu-Uganda. It was from there that I began to think of writing a book. I wanted to write a book titled *All Acholi Traditional Names Have Meanings*. In this book, I wanted to explain the meaning of Acoli names like Okeny, Onen, Opiyo, Acen, Olum, Oryiem, Acayo, Abalo, Akwero, Onek and many others that I cannot list all here. I found that I had a lot of academic work, so I suspended the writing project because I wanted to score high marks at the seminary.

In 1973, when the Government of Sudan and the leaders of Anya-nya One rebel group signed a peace deal at Adiss Ababa in Ethiopia, Bishop of Sudan said that all Sudanese seminarians who were in Uganda should go back to Sudan. In 1973 I started studying Philosophy in *Juba St Paul National Major Seminary*. Father Joseph Nyekindi, who later became a Bishop of Yambio, was a Rector. I completed Philosophy in 1975, and in 1976 I joined *St Paul National Seminary* in *Bussere National Major Seminary*, where I studied Theology. Eventually, I discovered that academic victory was not in the class-room because we were only three theologians in the class. For this reason, we wrote to the Bishops to allow us to study at *St. Thomas Aquinas National Major Seminary* in Kenya. Unfortunately, the lecturers at Bussere National Major Seminary were Italian and American fathers. They looked at our request as disrepute to them. One evening the fathers talked this issue over their supper. They said I was the one who enticed the other two students to think of going to study at St. Thomas Aquinas National Major Seminary. As a result, they resolved and sent me on a one year probation. Bishop Gabriel Ziber, who headed Wau Diocese, came to the Seminary to investigate the matter. He found out that I was innocent. He then asked the lecturers if they could allow me to resume studies at Bussere. Unfortunately, none of the lecturers agreed with the Bishop. In 1977 they sent me on the one year probation in Juba so that I could stay out of the seminary. When I was on probation, I asked Bishop Ereneo Dut of Juba Diocese if I could look for a job so that I could take care of my welfare before going back to the seminary. He did not object to my request. I was employed in the Ministry of Finance as an Office Clerk.

I worked in the Ministry of Finance for six months before the government appointed me Community Development Officer in the Regional Ministry of Cooperative and Community Development. The government transferred me to Torit District where I lived with Father Julius Igaa in *Torit Mission*. The one year probation elapsed but the Rector of Bussere National Seminary did not call me back to the Seminary. Subsequent to this, I left Torit Mission and rented a house in Malakia. In 1978, I married my senior wife, Mrs. Margarete Ayaa of Oruku (Madi). In December 1978, God blessed us with a child whom we named Emmanuel Onen (which means, behold God is with us). I served in Torit from 1978- to 1982, and then the government sent me back to Juba as Assistant Director of Community Development. In that year, *Agency for Cooperation and Research Development* (ACORD) began to work in partnership with Department of Community Development. The government saw my efficiency at work and promoted me to Coordinator of Community Development Support Unit where I supervised Community Officers of Equatoria Region, Upper Nile Region and Bahr El Ghazal Region.

In 1986 I started writing the book, *The History and Expressive Cultures of the Acholi of South Sudan*. The Dr. John Garang de Mabior, insurgency did not give me time to visit Acholi informants in different places. In 1990, when I was piecing up my work, my Uncle (my father's brother), Justice John Onge Kassiba observed that the book I was writing "would be useful to future generations." unfortunately, I did not know where I could get the money to publish the book.

In 1991 when the war in Juba intensified, I took refuge in Khartoum together with my family. Because of my good work record and efficiency CONCERN SUDAN (Irish International Organisation) employed me as a Refugee Program

Manager at Kosti where I worked from 1991 to 1994. Unfortunately, before I finished writing the book, my wife, Mrs. Margarete Ayaa passed away in 1993 from Kosti. I had five children with her one daughter and four sons. But one of the sons called John Onge, later died from Juba. My second wife Santa Alal was in Juba, South Sudfan, when we were in Kosti. In 1996 I went to Khartoum, and worked as Logistic Assistant Officer with Action Contra La Faim (ACF) at Jaborona Regugee Camps in Omdurman. In 1996 I married the third wife, Mrs. Faima Doka. I had the first child with her and called her Anna Achiro Olaa. In 1999 I went to study Diploma Primary Health Care at Halliah University Omdurman.

In 2001, the security situation in Khartoum grew tense. The soldiers of President Omer El Bashir were secretly killing them. Many people lost their lives. I then fled to Cairo-Egypt. Before I reached Cairo, I thought Cairo would be a resting place, but when I reached there I found life in Cairo as hard as sitting on fire. Sudanese traveled fearfully. Refugees slept in fear. The Egyptians stated calling us *Chokoleta*. Egyptians also increased rent for Sudanese refugees up to LS 500 for a three room house. Yet an Egyptian rented it at only Ls 20 to 30. In addition to that, most UNHCR workers were Egyptians. As a result, passing interviews in the office of UNHCR became very hard for Sudanese refugees. To get out of Egypt, refugees must for the decision of UNHCR for two or seven years. If they allowed you to go, they conditioned you to go to America, Canada, Finland, and Australia. Some Sudanese have never got their way out of Egypt. Some people went back to Sudan, but those who realised that there was no peace in Sudan are still in Egypt.

In 2003 I came to Australia, and I thought it would be easy for me to get a job here because of my vast experience. Unfortunately, Australian government did not recognise degrees of Sudanese universities. This made it a little difficult for me to get a job here. In 2004 I began to study Community Development in Dandenong TAFE, and graduated with Diploma in Community Development in 2005. From 2006 to 2008, I obtained B.A. in Human Services, Victoria University. When I was studying at Victoria University, I worked with Migrant Information Centre, Eastern Melbourne, on the terms of three days a week. On completion of the course, the Manager of Migrant Information Centre gave me Case Management job which was on the basis of five days per week. Although most of the employees of Migrant Information Centre were women, there was high level of solidarity among them. This made my work at Migrant Information Centre easy. When I was searching for other jobs from the Internet, I discovered that most employers wanted people with Master Degree. For this reason, I began to pursue Master in International Development at RMIT University-Melbourne campus. I completed this course in 2012 since I was a part time student and, at the same time, working to support my children.

In 2010, when I was sending the manuscript of *The History and Expressive Cultures of the Acholi of South Sudan* to Mwaka Emmanuel Lutukumoi in Uganda, I thought of writing another book in English. It is titled *The Short Social Anthropology of the Northern Luo of South Sudan*. Today I am writing my third book entitled *Money, Gifts and Sex: A sugar daddy and sugar baby in a new dress among African Australians*.

Introduction

First and foremost, I want to make it abundantly clear to readers that the title of this book suggests that some African Australians are deeply involved in "sugar" relationships. A sugar daddy indirectly pays money in exchange for sex, although not in the same way men pay cash money to sex workers. Although the African women, who are involved in sugar relationships, are not directly called sex workers, nevertheless they are really sex workers under the carpet. The difference between African sugar babies and other Australian sex workers lies in this that the African women do not receive cash soon after sexual intercourse as do other Australian sex workers. They receive their payments in the form of monthly or fortnightly allowances.

It is reported that back in Africa, and on arrival in Australia, marriage had been considered as the basis for household formation, production, and the means by which men and women gain access to a strong family fund. This is true because marriage constitutes an advantageous form of cooperation between a man and a woman, which works as a safety insurance for the family.

As the years passed by, life in their new country has impacted on the African Australians, and they misconceive the biblical principles and the Gospel teachings at large. As a result, they think of their material life first, and the teachings of the Holy Bible have become second.

Subsequently, some of the African Australians have failed to understand and apply the teachings of the Gospel into their daily lives. They have failed to understand that marriage is a covenant, a promise and commitment between husband and wife. Malachi 2:4, says, *"The Lord is witness between a husband and a wife"*. Mathew 19:3-6 tells us how the Pharisees were testing Jesus, when they said, *"Is it lawful to divorce one's wife for any cause?"* Jesus answered wonderfully, *"Have you not read that He who created them from the beginning made them male and female? Therefore, a man shall leave his father and his mother and hold fast to his wife, and the two shall become one flesh. So, they are no longer two but one flesh. What God has joined together, let not man separate"*. Ephesians 5:22-31 tells us further saying, *"Wives, submit to your own husband, as to the Lord ... Husbands love your wives, as Christ loved the church and gave himself up for her.... In the same way husbands should love their wives as their own bodies. He who loves his wife loves himself.... Therefore, a man shall leave his father and mother and hold fast to his wife and the two shall become one flesh"*. But today, some of the African Australians have changed the context of God to fit their worldly lives.

In this book, Saturnino Onyala discusses the hidden sugar relationships or what I called "under the carpet movement of sugar relationships among the African Australians". It is time for us to call a spade, a spade, because the acts are degrading our African cultures.

The practices of sugar relationships amongst African Australians have never been studied, although these practices are now in full swing.

This book begins by examining the general background to sugar relations in Australia, before and after the coming of the Africans, and sugar relationships in depth in Chapter 1. In addition, the author attempts to answer one of the burning questions, "Why some African Australians have become sugar daddies and sugar babies". There is no straightforward answer to this question, but the author tries to answer it anyway.

The African Australians who are involved in sugar relationships, do not want other people to know that they are in sugar relationships. For this reason, they have developed new terminology for "sugar daddy" and "sugar baby". As we shall see later in the book, the Africans have deliberately changed the term sugar daddy to brother or uncle and the term sugar baby to sister. This is what

I meant by saying, "A sugar daddy and sugar baby in a new dress among the African Australians".

Before starting to write this book, it was discovered that the topic for the book is sensitive because the people involved don't want to speak about it.

The book examines the financial side of being a single mother, and research revealed that some African women in Australia are enduring financial instability after divorce or separation. They find it difficult to feed themselves as well as their children, if they have any. We could call this "food insecurity". Not only this, they also endure the pressures and stress that come about as a result of divorce and separation.

Unlike back in Africa, here some women are working but although they are employed, they still find it difficult to make ends meet. The minimum wage available to single mothers is often not enough to meet the basic needs. As a result, they are forced to become sugar babies to support themselves financially. Some of the African women begin to sell sex to African men in motels, the sugar daddy's house, the sugar baby's home or in friends' homes. Therefore, sex sales among Africans is booming in Australia. It appears some women even look for a white sugar daddy.

Today, the modern form of sex selling is known as "sugar dating". In an African context, sugar dating is described differently from the Western sugar dating. From the African prospective, sugar dating is described as "relationships based on making money without any written contract or agreement in which the expectations of both man and woman would be made explicit". Study shows that it is the Anglo-Australians who make written agreements when sugar dating. A sugar baby can never slack off if she wants the relationship to last for many years.

The research found that among the African Australians, "a sugar daddy" or "brother/uncle" is defined as "a working man with reasonable income who has capacity to provide a financial allowance in exchange for sexual services".

The practices of sugar relationships have become increasingly popular among African communities in Australia; this appears to be due to the current economic conditions facing women in their new country. Research also revealed that some African women are utilizing dating (getting a brother/uncle) for financial purposes, while they move on with their daily family life.

Finding a sugar daddy for money is considerably stigmatizing and is often regarded as an indirect form of prostitution. This book, therefore, attempts to identify ways the African men endorse and market themselves to the women.

The book also attempts to identify possible places African men and women would use to advertise themselves. Onyala went further to describe African Australians' background in Chapter 2 and how they become involve in the development and promotion of sugar relationships. He identifies the best cities for Anglo-Australians to find their sugar daddies and sugar babies and also examines the skills stream and Australian's official Humanitarian Migration Programmes.

The book explores why some married men and women are involved in sugar relationships. The book goes on to examine how some African men and women are involved in multiple sugar daddies.

Chapter 4 identifies and discusses ways women have chosen to have multiple sugar daddies and describes the positive and negative sides of both men and women, including single fathers and single mothers.

Subsequently, the book seeks to critically examine the techniques used by sugar daddies to entice single mothers and some housewives.

Literature pertaining to African sugar relationships is not available, and as such it becomes difficult to find references. There is a great need for professionals to have an awareness of the social implications of sugar relationships, which could include physical, psychological and emotional risks involved in this practice of dating among the African Australians.

The author thinks that by disclosing the facts about sugar relationships, this will help family support workers, psychologists, and social workers to assist African Australians, who are involved or are becoming involved in sugar relationships, to sort out or to avoid entering into the potential problems.

In the research conducted, it was revealed that there was no indication that sugar relationships among African Australians would end up in marriage, but some people expected that this could be a possibility; but it is more likely that a sugar baby with multi-relationships would not get married. This topic is discussed more in depth in Chapter 6 of this book.

As mentioned before, it is imperative for African Australians to know what the potential effect of marketing sex could bring on them. This is crucial, and the book explores the risks involved with sugar relationships. The book also explores how the body of a man and woman works.

Onyala believes that the implications of the findings in this book are important tools for social service providers, counsellors, family support workers, psychologists and students of arts and social science.

Chapter One
Information Background

Background to the sugar daddy
and sugar baby culture in Australia

The invention of the term 'sugar daddy' in the Western World can be traced to 1925 in America by a businessman (a chocolate salesman) called Robert Welch (1899-1985) and which later spread to other parts of the world in about the 1990s. In the beginning, the term sugar daddy was known as "Papa-Sucker", and in 1932 the name become known as sugar daddy, and this led to the introduction of sugar babies in 1935. In 2006, a businessman called Branden Wade launched the Seeking Arrangement website in order to serve as a sort of digital matchmaker. The site now has over 3 million users worldwide, and its numbers are growing daily. A report says that the majority of users of Seeking Arrangement are females.

However, the origin of sugar daddy remains obscure. Some people think the term sugar daddy might have stemmed from the 1908 marriage between Adolph Spreckels, an American heir to a sugar fortune, with a woman 24 years old his junior. His wife, Alma de Breltville called him a sugar daddy. According to Sarah Daly (2017) the term "a sugar baby" which was known as "a kept woman" suggests a person who is maintained in a comfortable lifestyle by a rich man so that she would be available for his sexual pleasure any time he needs her.

Study shows that Australia is one of the counties in the world with a growing population of sugar daddies. Thus, a dating site for sugar daddies and sugar babies was founded in Australia in 2001. Australians found it easier to arrange dating through a dating site rather than face-to-face or by mail. According to the Canberra Times in 2018, there were 82,760 sugar babies registered for membership and by the year 2016 the memberships went up to 425,761. The report also revealed that the growth from 2016 to 2018 was five times, and this was driven by university students. It was reported by a dating Australian website spokesperson, that students were increasingly seeking alternative methods to offset the financial pressures of university, as the average cost of a degree in Australia was rising to almost $30,000 in the year 2018. It is reported that some students who have become sugar babies only want money and expensive gifts, but do not want sexual intercourse. As a result, one sugar daddy told his sugar baby, "If you are not ready to have sex with me, then don't go on the website because you're pretty much putting yourself in that situation". Eventually, a sugar baby ended up asking for money, as the Seeking Arrangement website is for selling happiness and not a fantasy.

Seeking Arrangement founder Brandon Wade says, "I am not selling a fantasy. I think at the end of the day I'm selling happiness. I'm selling the fact that life is really short, and we're all on Earth for a reason. We want to be happy. For some it is about finding love and romance in a way that makes them happy. For others, it's to be surrounded by three, or five, or ten beautiful women." (Source 60 Minutes, Channel 9.)

However, some universities like Canberra University, denied the allegation made by the dating site spokesperson that university students were increasingly seeking alternative methods to offset the financial pressures of university on them. They said they are not aware of their students being involved in Seeking Arrangement. But the 60 Minutes program on Channel 9 revealed that Seeking Arrangement released its list of "Fastest Growing Sugar Baby Schools" in March 2019 stating that Monash University came out on top with 209 new sign-ups last year, followed by RMIT with 184, University of Sydney with 170 and University of Melbourne with 128. With the list, the site also claimed more than 177,000 of its 20 million members are Australian university students.

The bottom-line is that it appears there are more than 200,000 sugar daddies and sugar babies in Australia. According to statistical records, there are currently more than 17, 000 sugar daddies in the country, these are the people who have taken to the internet and dating sites to find love and date. Subsequently, from this record we could conclude that out of the 200,000 sugar relationship participants, 91.5 percent of them are sugar babies and only 8.5 percent are sugar daddies. This tells us that in Australia there are more women in the sugar relationships than men.

However, it is reported that the largest population of sugar daddies and sugar babies in the world are found in the United States of America, followed by Canada, United Kingdom, Australia, and Colombia.

In Australia and other countries in the Western World, sugar daddy and sugar baby relationships are considered normal, it is not about prostitution or escorts; it is accepted as something legal. They asserted that prostitution is about reaching a specific agreement to exchange cash or material possessions for sex.

Interestingly, in Australia and other regions in developed countries, a sugar baby can be a female or a male looking for a successful and generous relationship. They seek chances to upgrade their lifestyle. However, most sugar babies are identified as females, who are seeking heterosexual relationships with male sugar daddies.

When I was doing my research, I discovered that there are some cities in Australia where sugar babies can easily find their sugar daddies. We shall discuss this later in this chapter.

According to Seeking Arrangement's statistics, the average age of a sugar daddy in Australia, ranges between 39 — 70 years old and such men, by definition, must earn between AUD $230,000 and $250,000 annually. These men usually secure in their future financially because of the large amount of annual income they receive. For men of these ages, especially those who have been through a divorce or have never had the time to settle down, this would now be the best time for them to look for companionship with women who are generally younger than them.

It is reported that from the annual income of $230,000 — $250, 000, a sugar daddy spends around $2,800 — $4,000 a month on a sugar baby. It is also said that from the amount a sugar baby receives, and if a sugar baby is a student, she will use 36% of the money to pay tuition fees, 23% of the money to pay rent, and the remaining 41% is used for food, clothes, bills and medication.

What interested me most in this study is that I discovered sugar babies are receiving payments from their sugar daddies just for personal interests. As a result, they must be ready 24 hours a day and 7 days a week to never say "No" to any request a sugar daddy may ask to be performed. Here I can see problems arising with sugar babies who have multiple sugar daddies, (we shall discuss a sugar baby with multiple sugar daddies later in Chapter 4). According to Dr Kyle Livie (2019) the phenomenon of men with power and money using those aspects to attract women is certainly not new. By the end of the 19th century, a phenomenon known as "treating" began to arise, in which shop-girls and other unmarried women with low-paying jobs relied upon men to provide them with money for housing, dinners, bills, etc in exchange for being an escort. SugarDaddyMeet (2009) reported that in the 1960s the number of sugar daddies was relatively low in Australia, but with acceptance of the practice in society, it appears that numbers are steadily starting to rise.

We have just discussed above about rich older men seeking companionship of younger women. There are many reasons which would lead such men to look for relationships. One of the reasons is that older rich men enjoy many perks in life, which their future has provided for them. They usually enjoy having young women around them and want the young women to be part of their lives.

Interestingly, it is said that a number of married sugar daddies are joining the group, although it is reported that in the last six years their number has dropped from 65 percent in 2013 to 29 percent in 2019. This literarily means that the lifestyle is heavily accepted by single men. The study also suggested that a good number of married Australian men are sugar daddies.

Study shows that there are nearly 120,000 young Anglo-Australian women who have turned to wealthy older Anglo-Australian men to pay for their lavish lifestyle, school fees for children, and daily expenses in exchange of companionship.

Globally, there are two types of sugar daddy relationships: the first type is known as a long-term relationship; the second type is known as a short-term transactional relationship. Experiences tell us that some men with a long-term relationship find it difficult to maintain "status quo" because at the end of the day, they realise that it is unreasonable, as it requires more time to be spent with a sugar baby. Subsequently, a good number of Australian sugar daddies prefer to practise short-term sugar relationships.

More importantly, in Australia every sugar baby wants her own successful "quid pro" where they loan their beauty, sham and youthful energy for money. Some sugar babies even like touring the country or travelling overseas with a sugar daddy. One of the other things that struck me during my research, is that I thought sugar relationships could lead to marriages, but I discovered that a single sugar daddy usually tells their partner from the beginning of their first meeting that "marriage and children are never going to happen". In such a situation, a sugar daddy becomes a mentor, teacher, protector and lover of the sugar baby.

The best cities to meet a sugar daddy in Australia

When I first arrived in Australia in 2003, and when I heard of the practices of sugar daddies and sugar babies, I thought that these practices were being done in one or two cities. As time passed by, it became clear to me that sugar daddy and sugar baby relationships are being practised in all the capital cities of Australia, with exception of Darwin. A large number of women working as sugar babies in Australia admit they do it to help them pay bills. In this book, I have identified six cities in the country, where those interested persons can meet sugar daddies. According to the records, found on various dating sites, it appears the top six sugar daddy capital cities are the following:-

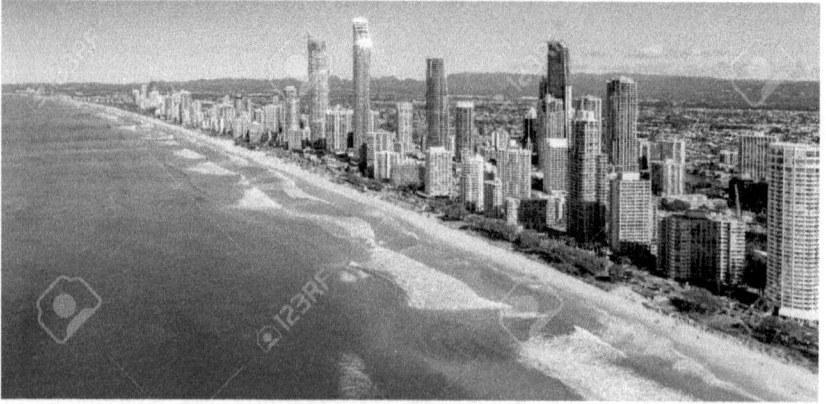

Figure: 1. Gold Coast

▸ Brisbane: Records show that many rich and successful men are found in Brisbane; it is reported that the Gold Coast has the highest population of sugar daddies in the State, with a ratio of nearly 4 men out of 100 qualifying as a sugar daddy. This explains why many young Australian women are relocating to the Gold Coast, because this is a place where a lady can easily find a sugar daddy. From the records we learn that Sydney comes next after Brisbane.

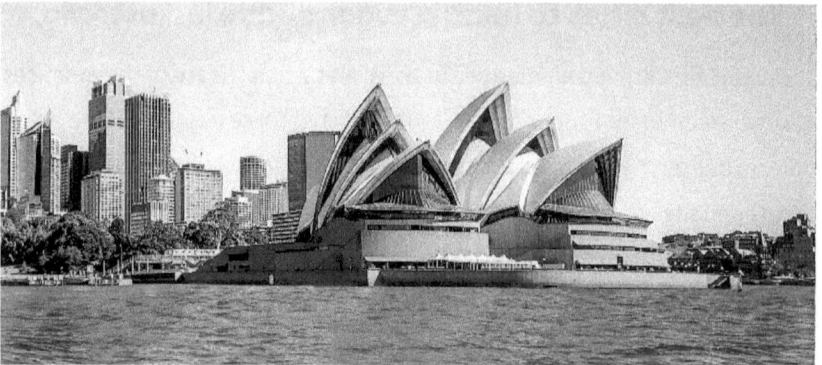

Figure: 2, Sydney

▸ Sydney: Although Sydney does not have the highest population of sugar daddies like Brisbane, nevertheless, the active nightlife in the city makes it more likely to have a good ratio of sugar daddies. Mr Wade told 60 Minutes that in Sydney there was a woman who has had $150,000 spent on her by wealthy married men; and he is continuously encouraging women on his website to look for sugar daddies. He is telling women that if they are poor and they are constantly hanging out with the poor, they're never going to find opportunities in life. Subsequently, he is directing women to his website for marketing. From this short narrative you can understand how popular a sugar relationship is in Sydney in particular and in Australia in general.

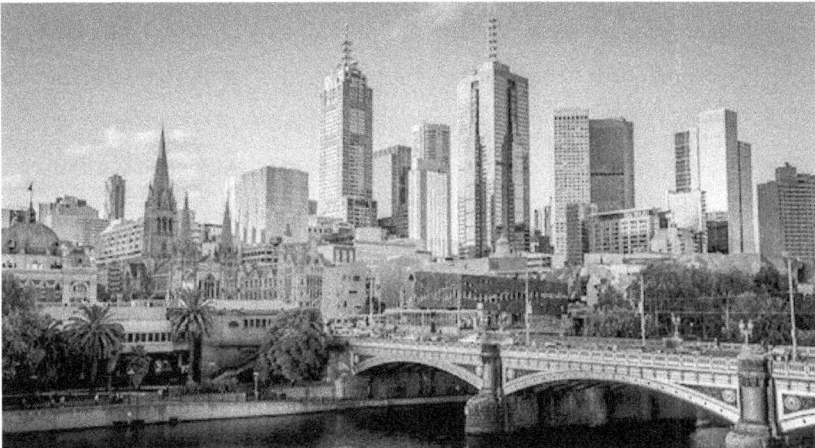

Figure: 3. Melbourne's Yarra River

▶ Melbourne: This city is constantly growing and changing, which makes it the perfect place to find wealthy men who are seeking younger women for companionship or sex. There are many stories which could be told about Melbourne but due to time and lack of space in this book, I cannot narrate all of them. However, I am going to tell one true story told by a sugar baby who is a student in Melbourne. Because of confidentiality, I am not going to name the of a student, nor am I going to name the university where she was studying. The student from University-x said, "I earned US$50,000 from a series of wealthy men as a sugar baby. I declared that without this money I wouldn't have been able to afford my rent and university fees. Currently, I am studying while working full-time. I am 26 years old and earns AUD$60,000 per year; I pay $1,800 a month in rent. Being an overseas student, I pay upfront fees of between $8,500 and $10,000 per semester". Another student from Melbourne University also said, "The arrangement helps me survive through university. I have learnt that, what I was making in two weeks working in hospitality, now I can make it in about three to four hours on a date".

Due to pressing financial difficulties, this student from Melbourne University has used the controversial sugar dating website Seeking Agreement to connect with rich men that could support her financially. She was able to connect with some wealthy men, who lavished her with expensive meals and clothing, allowances and even holidays. (Source: amp.news.com.au, 2019).

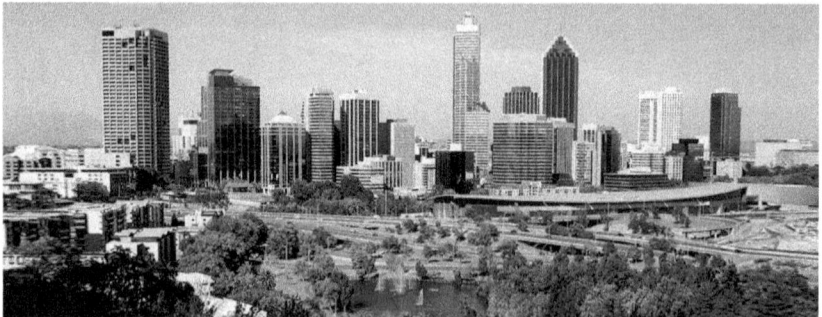

Figure: 4. Perth City

▶ Perth: According to the report, Melbourne is followed by Perth. The common website women in Perth use to find a sugar daddy is SugardaddyPerth.com.au. The West Coast of Australia is attracting new interest when it comes to finding a sugar daddy or sugar baby. Many women are re-allocating themselves in Western Australia according to their interests and availability of sugar daddies. The record shows that Adelaide is the next city after Perth.

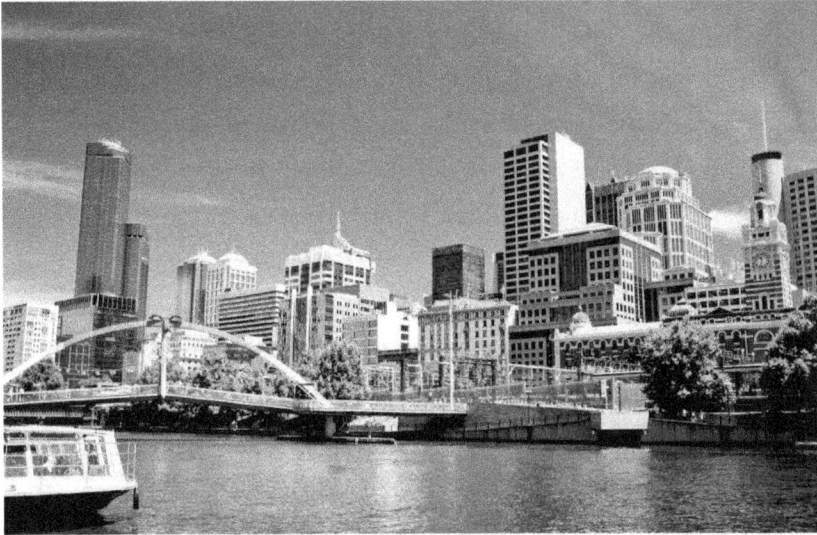

Figure: 5. Adelaide City

▶ Adelaide: It is reported that SugarDaddyAdelaide.com.au was founded in 2008. Many young women who are looking for a sugar daddy, use this dating site to find wealthy men of their dreams.

This website has been offering services to sugar daddies and sugar babies for more than eleven years. Like many cities in Australia, Adelaide is constantly growing and changing, especially being the South Australia's cosmopolitan coastal capital, where many governmental and financial institutions are emerging.

Adelaide ranks highly in terms of quality of life, being constantly listed in the world's top ten most liveable cities (out of 140 cities worldwide). It was also ranked the most liveable city in Australia by the Property Council of Australia in 2011, 2012 and 2013, and it appears many people have come to Adelaide from Darwin, Melbourne, Tasmania and Sydney.

▶ Canberra: Records shows that Canberra is the sixth city in Australia where sugar daddies are found in great number. Canberra is located between Sydney and Melbourne; its population is growing given the fact that it is currently Australia's capital city. As we mentioned in Melbourne, searching for a sugar daddy is not only the work of single and married women, studies show that female students from the universities are also deeply involved in the practice. According to the Canberra Times dated 28th October 2018, it was revealed that 106 female students studying in the universities around Canberra, as well as Canberra Institute of Technology, turned to sugar daddies to pay tuition fees and rent. The website developed for dating was challenged by many people as promoting prostitution in the society although this critic was denied by Kimberly de la Cruz, spokesperson of Seeking Arrangement.

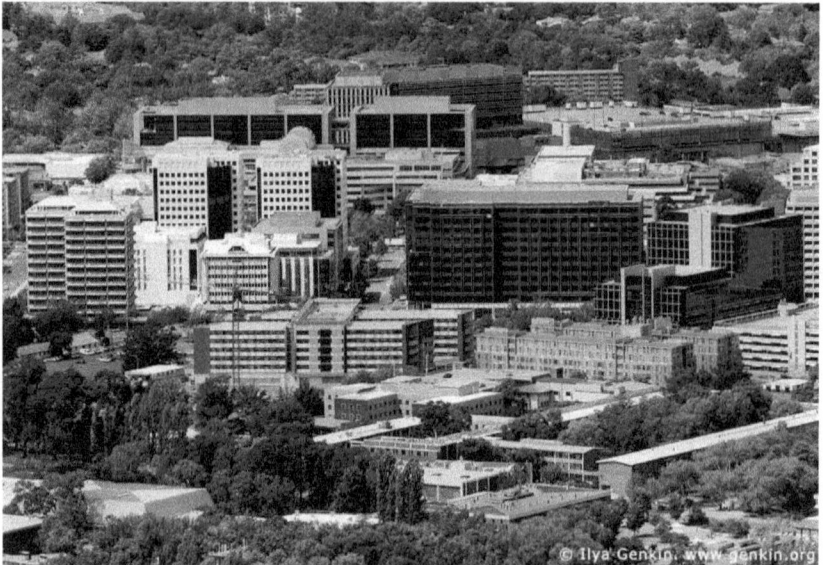

Figure: 6. Canberra View from Black Mountain Tower

Methods for getting a sugar daddy in Australia

It is believed that different women have different ways of getting a sugar daddy in Australia. I have learned from my research that there are two main ways; this can be "direct approach" or "indirect approach". To understand these two approaches, let me explain how they work. I will also try to explain how sugar babies get their allowances. I addition, I think it is important to understand how the people perceive a sugar daddy in Australia.

▶ Direct Approach — It is generally observed that a woman who is interested in finding a sugar daddy through a direct approach always asks the man directly. She can ask him by saying, "Have you ever had an arrangement before?" It is generally believed that a woman who wants to become a sugar baby is never afraid to ask such questions. She knows that if she does not ask, she will never get what she wants, since a sugar relationship is based on "give" and "take" exchange. So if a man answers "Yes" to her question above, this means the man is interested and the woman can begin to talk about allowances. In the course of discussions, the man would also ask the woman, "Have you had an arrangement before?" When a woman hears such a question, she usually feels trapped or pushed into a corner, so she thinks twice before she answers the question. However, if she wants her application to be accepted, she could answer "Yes". When a woman answers "Yes" to the man's question, this usually followed with the talk about the allowance she had in the past. The thing a woman should avoid in this conversation is that she must never tell the man about her previous sugar daddy's dark sides (e.g. I have had a sugar daddy, but he never gave allowances etc). It is reported that the main reason behind why a woman should keep this to herself at this stage is that if she starts to complain about her ex-sugar daddy, the new man may develop a negative attitude and may decide not to accept her application altogether. Therefore, we can say that using a direct approach is good, but one needs to be careful not to break the relationship with reckless words. The second way a woman can use to get a sugar daddy is called the "indirect approach".

▶ Indirect Approach: The indirect approach can be viewed as the art of communication between the parties, but sometimes the direct approach does not work for an individual to achieve her dream/goal. In this case a potential sugar baby may use an indirect approach, where she cannot use a direct statement such as "I want an allowance", but she could ask an indirect question by just saying, "Can we go shopping?" Alternatively, if the man is in good mood at the time, a woman could send text messages to his mobile telling him what types of dress, shoes, mobile or watch she likes. She might even tell him, "I cannot call because I have no credit". This is an indirect way to say that I want some money. In another way, a potential sugar baby could ask if the man could pay for her gym membership, or personal training sessions, because she wants to look slim and beautiful. When a man hears this, he may put his hand into his pockets and pull out some dollars and give her. However, one thing most of the potential African sugar babies fail to understand is that African sugar daddies are more willing to give money to a woman when he can see that he benefits from it. That is why an indirect approach works so well. A sugar baby should give time for a sugar daddy to develop a lasting interest in her, as a result, some of these men who are not prepared to become a long-term sugar daddy, often keep on moving from one sugar baby to another. But once a woman gives enough time for a man to develop an interest in her, the next time they go out for a coffee, she could use this opportunity to tell him what type of dresses she wants to wear or what type of things are currently on her priority list but that she cannot obtain them because of financial difficulty. Experience shows that once a man has developed a lasting interest in a woman, whenever he hears such indirect questions, he would immediately pull out cash from his wallet and give it to her.

▶ Payment Methods for the Allowances: There are many ways a sugar baby could receive allowances from a sugar daddy. However, the best and recommended way to receive money from a man is through cheque or cash in hand. A sugar baby should not allow her sugar daddy (brother/uncle) to give her money through her bank account. This is what some of the African women in Australia have failed to understand, so they give their account information to the men to deposit weekly or monthly allowances into. However it is better that they do not give this information to their sugar daddies, but receive cash or materials. It is recommended that a sugar baby should not reveal her bank account details or any personal information to her man, because she does not know him enough. Personal information is "owned" and should not be shared with a second or third party. Therefore, it is good to arrange to receive cash rather than a direct deposit, as this is the safest way to get allowances from a sugar daddy; although it may not be as convenient.

▶ How the People Perceive a Sugar Daddy in Australia: It is believed that more and more men are joining sugar daddy programmes in Australia. The majority of Australians perceive a sugar daddy to be a rich old man in a wheelchair. There is also a report that many ladies are dreaming of becoming a sugar baby to meet the wants of the rich old men. Australian women who want to become sugar babies believe that by doing so, they stand a better chance to enjoy the finer things in life; because a sugar daddy would offer these things. They also believe that a sugar daddy can help pay school fees — where appropriate, rent, bills and much more. With all those views in mind, we can conclude that a sugar daddy is always ready to take care of a sugar baby and ready to do everything for her at all cost.

Chapter Two
Background To African Australians

Migration of Africans to Australia

Australia has had a growing African community over the last thirty years; the African have migrated to Australia through the two routes as follows:

- Skills migration and family reunion programmes: The statistics from the Department of Immigration and Border Protection indicates that the Africans who have come through this channel are mainly people from Nigeria, Ghana, The Republic of Congo (Zaire), Zimbabwe, Kenya, Egypt, Mali and South African. The Skills Stream accounts for most African migrants to Australia, and this migration took place between 1985-2000 and 2001-2009. The records from the Department of Immigration show that 80,252 Africans migrated during these two periods. It is reported that over 90 percent of Skills Stream migrants have come from South and East Africa. The breakdown of some are as follows:
  - 50,914 Skills Stream migrants came from South Africa
  - 10,666 Skills Stream migrants came from Zimbabwe
  - 3,181 Skills Stream migrants came from Egypt
  - 8,500 Skills Stream migrants came from Kenya
  - 4,419 Skills Stream migrants came from Nigeria
  - 3,770 Skills Stream migrants came from Ghana

From the above statistics, we can conclude that South Africans are the majority of the Africans who live in Australia, followed by Zimbabweans, Kenyans, Nigerians, Ghana, with the Congolese appearing to be the minority. Since 2001 Skills migrants to Australia have been eligible to apply both onshore and offshore, however some of them came through sponsorship or an independent points-testing basis.

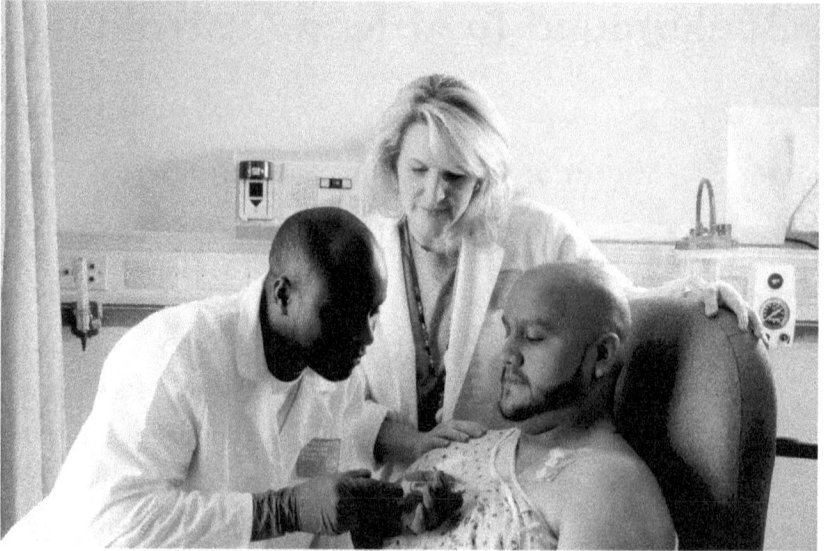

Figure: 7. African doctor with white doctor colleague.

The occupation groups within the Skills Stream were professionals, including medical doctors, nurses, accountants and university lecturers. However, records show that some of these professionals came to Australia for studies and their training was paid for by poor African countries; after graduation they are put to work in Australia. (Senator, Michael Forshaw, 2011, PP. 207-208)

In other words, offshore Skills Assessment is a pathway for applicants seeking permanent migration to Australia, for work in a nominated occupation and the holder of a passport from a nominated country. It is the responsibility of the applicant to contact the relevant assessment authority for their occupation and he/she will be given a skills assessment. Soon after this an applicant will have to do Skill Assessment tests, which are tests designed to help employers evaluate the skills of their job candidates and employees. Using Skills Assessment tests helps companies ensure that their job candidates, as well as their current employees, have the required skills to successfully perform their jobs.

Australia Humanitarian Programmes:

The other groups of Africans came to Australia through Australian Humanitarian Programmes. The people who came through this channel are from Sudan, South Sudan, Ethiopia, Eritrea, Somalia, Congo, Liberia, Chad, Uganda, Egypt and Rwanda.

Surprisingly, the number of African refugees who came in the same period (1985-2000 and 2001-2009) accounts for a far lower number, compared to the Skills Stream migrants who came in the same period.

The refugees came under two components of Australian's official Humanitarian Migration Programmes. One group came through offshore assessment, which is done in the Australian Embassy in a given country. The statistics show that about 70% of the African refugees came to Australia through offshore assessment.

Soon after this, an applicant will have to do Skill Assessment tests which are designed to help employers evaluate the skills of their job candidates and employees.

However, the statistics from the office of Department of immigration and Border Protection shows that about 30 percent of the African refugees came through onshore assessment.

Pathway to a sugar daddy and sugar baby

The experiences of the African community in Australia show us that for the first 3 — 5 years after arrival, men and women live happily with their wives and husbands; but as time passed by, some of them started learning the Western world way of life which is new to many. Subsequently, and prematurely, some Africans (especially women) started to abandon the good binding African cultures that could be used to build a family in the new country and preferred new cultures, without understanding what the consequences would be. Shortly, many of them started living with stress as a result of family violence, due to unnecessary fights and the rate of divorce grew higher.

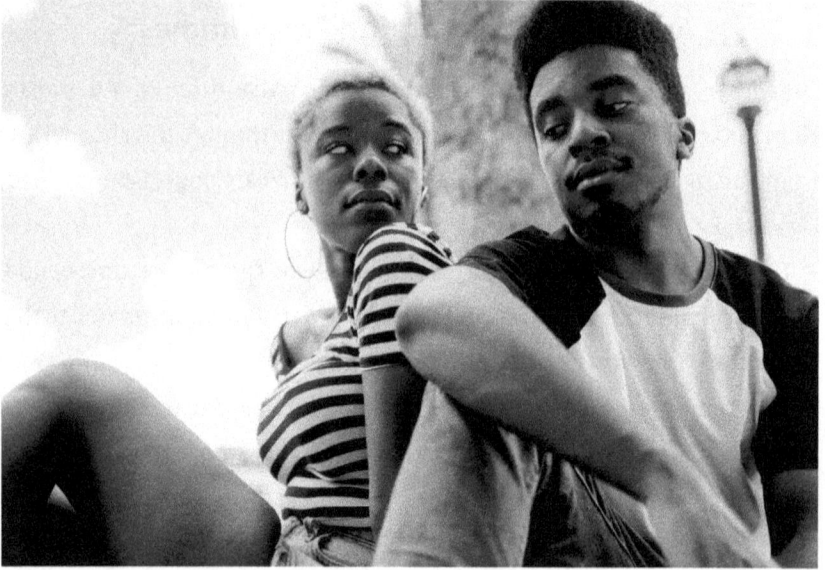

Figure: 8. Two cultures, resulting in family violence.

Many community organisations in Australia have documented family violence (FV) and the rate of divorce among the African Australians was going up in 2006, but unfortunately this information have never been published because of confidentiality and privacy rules. The reports revealed that the rate of family violence and divorce increased among the African families as they tried to settle in a new country. This creates room for single mothers and single fathers to do what they think best to promote their lifestyle. It also provides an opportunity for single mothers and single fathers to meet their unmet material and sexual needs.

Single mothers started to cultivate the need for expensive clothes, makeup, latest mobile phones and so on, to make them look beautiful in the eyes of hunting men. However, they did not have enough money to buy all these expensive items. This eventually led to the introduction of the sugar baby and sugar daddy culture among African Australians. Both African men and women know very well that such activity has a stigma attached to it, yet they think that the best way to avoid stigma is to keep the practices of sugar relationships top secrete -under the carpet by giving new names to the users. So they changed the term "sugar daddy" to "brother/uncle" and the term "sugar baby" to "sister". They have done this purposely to prevent other people from understanding what they are up to.

It is unfortunate that there has not been comprehensive research conducted on African Australian single mothers and housewives who became sugar babies, widows, as well as widowers, single fathers and married men who become sugar daddies. In the absence of this information, there is high need to study the population of Africans in Australia, to develop a general body of data on characteristics of African society.

Whether young or old, the Africans have been faced with two cultures in their new country; they have African cultures and Australian cultures and as a result, many Africans are trapped between these two cultures and do not know which to follow. It is paramount to know that Africans are coming from a patriarchal society where the husband is considered to be the head of the home, and the woman is considered a minister of finance and source of productions. Some people say a man is "a head" and a woman is "a neck" in family life.

Africans are proud of their family structure; back in African a husband comes first, a wife comes second, and a child comes third. Dogs do not figure in African family structure, and as such they are not counted. Unfortunately, Australian culture has turned the African family structure upside down. Here in Australia the law puts a child first, a wife comes second, a dog comes third, and the husband (man) comes fourth or last in the new family restructure. This family restructure reduces husbands or men to nothing in the eyes of society which often leads to stress and mental health among African men.

However, to some African women, the new family restructure is good, because they think that assimilation into Australian culture means changing your fundamental cultures. In other words, they assume that assimilating into Australian culture means dropping all their cultures, whether it be a good or a bad one. Experiences show us that this misunderstanding often leads to depression and occasionally has led to suicide.

The bottom-line is that assimilation does not mean dropping your cultures completely, rather it means dropping what are not accepted in Australian culture and keeping what is acceptable. Australia is a multicultural society where some people, like Greek, Italians, are keeping parts of their good culture. So why don't African Australians do the same?

Therefore, misunderstanding of "assimilation" into Australian culture and the restructure of family have led some African Australians to divorce, and that in turn has led them to become sugar babies and sugar daddies. Many African men and women are not prepared to become sugar daddies and sugar babies, and they even failed to understand that sugar relationships go with responsibilities. Providing financial assistance to a sugar baby becomes the primary responsibility of the African sugar daddy, which eventually leads to the cutting down of the family budget (if a man is married). Subsequently, there will not be enough money to support the family and not enough money available to send overseas to relatives, who need financial support from their relatives in Australia.

Last but not least, the cost of living in Australia is relatively high, and for a man (sugar daddy or brother/uncle) to make their sugar relationship last longer, he will have to struggle to provide a sugar baby (sister) with enough and appropriate financial support. If the man is a married sugar daddy, this will always lead to family problems, because the man would not know how much money is "considered sufficient and appropriate" for a sugar baby.

In Chapter 1, we have discussed that among Anglo-Australians, a sugar baby can be female or male, but it is not true for African Australians, they do not recognise a male as a sugar baby; among the Africans, sugar babies are only identified as females and all are seeking heterosexual relationships with male sugar daddies. So, my study and research focus is on the experiences of this numerically dominant group.

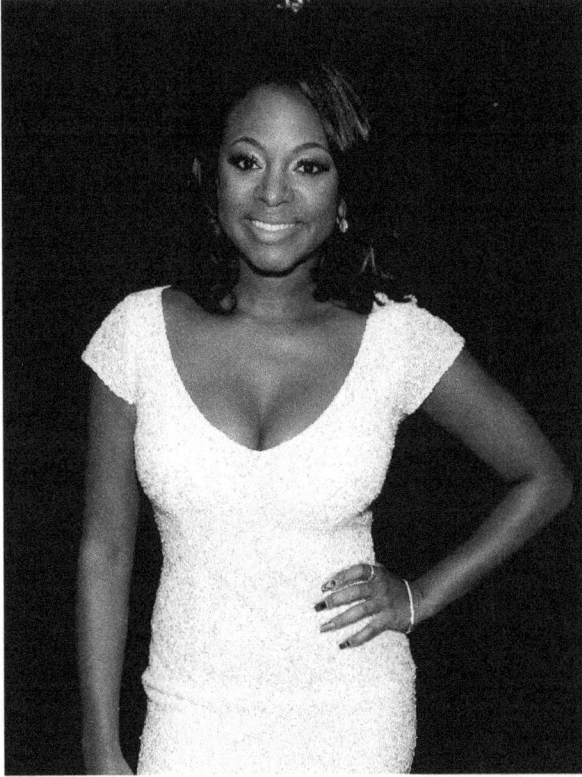

Figure: 9. A typical African Sugar Baby

For some women, being a sugar baby is a lifetime commitment but for others, it is something they do for a while to get them to the next step of life

Chapter Three
A Sugar Daddy and Sugar Baby

An African sugar daddy operates
on a different platform

A study shows that Anglo-Australian sugar daddies and sugar babies operate on different platforms from that of African Australian sugar daddies and sugar babies. According to Anglo-Australians, an agreement must be first reached between a sugar daddy and a sugar baby, before involving gifts and sex. In the agreement a sugar daddy may agree to pay rent for a sugar baby's current property. However, the agreement reached does not include other things, which are usually covered by allowances. Although a sugar daddy and sugar baby may have reached an agreement, they don't make an agreement for an allowance — it is open and there is no clarity on how much a sugar daddy is expected to give to the woman; similarly, it is not clear on what a man expects to get in return from the woman. As a result, a sugar daddy is often left wondering "how much is too much" regarding the services that a sugar baby provides.

Moreover, among the African Australians, agreement is never reached between the participants. One of my informants told me that one reason why African Australian sugar daddies and sugar babies do not make an agreement is that African sugar babies expect more and more financial support from the poor men who have insufficient income; the woman assumes that an agreement may interrupt or restrict the flow of money from the sugar daddy's wallet into her wallet. Therefore, most African sugar babies think that if such an agreement is done, it may close the "supply doors". One woman jokingly said, "When an allowance agreement is not reached between the sugar daddy and sugar baby, this gives an opportunity for a sugar baby to ask for more and more financial support, and in this way, a woman will be committed to the demands of the man (sugar daddy or brother)".

Another reason I have discovered in my research as to why the African Australians do not make an agreement is that sugar daddies (brothers) are not always ready to pay the full rent for African sugar babies (sisters). However, there is the possibility that an African sugar daddy could contribute some cash to meet part of the rent, but not the full amount. As I mentioned above, African Australian sugar daddies cannot commit themselves to this agreement because of the low pay they receive from their employers. And for the married sugar daddies, they cannot do it firstly because of their low income and secondly because of the roles and responsibilities they have in their families.

In Chapter 1, we have made it clear that the annual income of an Anglo-Australian man, who is defined as a sugar daddy, ranges between AUD $230,000 and $250,000 per year. Research reveals that African Australian sugar daddies' annual incomes are far below Anglo-Australians' incomes; African Australian incomes range between AUD $50,000 and $200,000 per annum and from this amount, a man (brother) spends around $300 to $1,500 a month on his sugar baby (sister). Therefore, this is the amount the African Australians consider enough and appropriate to support a sugar baby per calendar month.

However, some African Australian sugar babies would like men (brothers/ uncles) to spend more than $1,500; without understanding that "frog jumps according to its power". During my conversation with one of the African men (name confidential) he told me, "If my sugar baby is available every time I want her for sex, I will increase her payment or allowance, but if she is on and off in my sexual demands, I will not increase the monthly payment". From this narrative, we can understand that if an African man gives a sugar baby $300 per month, and a sugar baby response timely to his demands, he will increase the monthly allowance from $300 to $500 or more. In other words, we can say that the more a sugar daddy continues to increase monthly allowance, the more a sugar baby is expected to keep the appointments -to be available at all time for services.

One of the women said to me in a conversation, "If a sugar daddy does not increase the monthly allowance as I expect, why should I stick to our appointments or respect the appointments — good service demands sufficient financial increase and more money means regular services. In this way I would be happy and attractive to him".

It is believed that those African women who have become sugar babies, believe beyond doubt that the African men will provide them with an opportunity to enjoy the finer things, which other African women, who are not sugar babies, do not have. For this reason, one of African women told me in an informal conversation, "If I have a sugar daddy who provides me with everything I need, I can take care of him properly. And if the sugar daddy is a married man, I can take care of him more than his wife. I will give him special food that he does not eat in his house and above all I will treat him like a baby".

When I heard this, I pondered why women who become sugar babies expect married men to service them better than their wives and children! I was also surprised and shocked by the above statement from the woman. I thought that such a woman is more financial support; she may demand more fund from the man, and it is this fund can only encourage her to provide services to him. It is generally believed that such a man would expect the man to provide her, in addition, with quality shoes, handbags, clothes, earrings etc. and where possible the man could even pay part of her bills.

As I mentioned earlier in this book, African Australian sugar daddies are not usually ready to spend too much money on the endless wants of a sugar baby. Instead, they look more on how much a sugar baby responds to their demands, that is, they want to balance the scale of give and take.

Interestingly, the study also found that most of African sugar babies in Australia, are shy to talk about compensation and remuneration. On one hand they are shy because they think that if they talk about compensation to their men (brothers/uncles) it would look awkward -it is not good to bring up such a sensitive topic with someone you are interested in. On the other hand, they think that discussing about the increase of an allowance may block their way for more demands. The reality is that most of the African sugar daddies have realised that providing sugar babies with money on a 'per need" basis is not good enough, because this would result in constantly requesting more and more. And many of African sugar daddies begin to feel that some of the sugar babies are demanding too much.

More importantly, some of the African women have begun to ask their sugar daddies to build for their parents the modern houses in Africa.

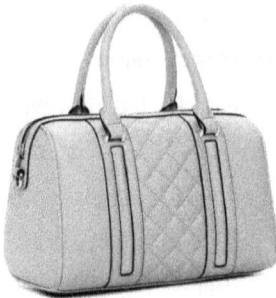

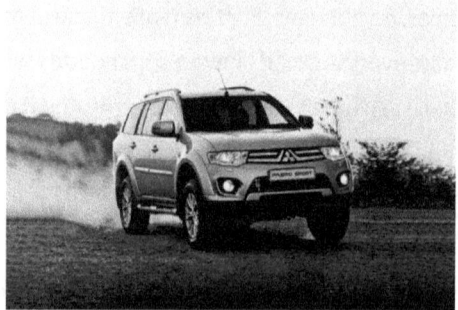

Figure: 10. Some requests of the sugar baby

These expenses often raise the eyebrows of men, they feel that these unnecessary expenses are degrading the meaning of a sugar daddy. According to the African sugar daddies, they think that they should rather give money freely to a sugar baby -a gift should be done at the wish of a man. For this reason, men don't want women to take advantage of financial assistance they give them and use it as an opportunity to exploit men. According to many men, they think that what they give allowances to sugar babies is enough, and they do not want more pressure put on them, for otherwise they walk away from the relationship. It is believed that men are thinking this way, because they find it difficult to keep track of how much money they spent on sugar baby.

I do not want to emphasize in this book that an African sugar daddy does not want to keep record of what he is giving to his sugar baby in exchange for sex and mutual relationship. Although study shows that the practice of a sugar daddy and sugar baby is not something new for the Africans. Back in Africa, sugar relationships are common, and the practices spread across the continent. However, some African men argue that although a sugar relationship is not something new to the Africans, the practice of sugar relationships among the Africans in Australia still has many problems. Some African men advocate that the practice of sugar relationships should be discouraged and to accomplish this in Australia. They wish that a strong campaign should be conducted. And this campaign should be aimed to discourage women from becoming sugar babies; because if women stop becoming sugar babies, this automatically would mean that men can drop the idea of having sugar babies as there would be no women in the market for the purpose. Philosophically speaking, to have something, it must exist. So instead of directing the campaign towards women alone, the other campaign should be directed towards irresponsible African Australian men (sugar daddies). In this campaign sugar daddies should be condemned by all members of African communities in Australia. This sounds good in theory, but it may not be possible for two main reasons. Firstly, it is difficult to identify African sugar daddies to be challenged and condemned. Secondly, it is impossible to do this because sugar relationships among the African communities are been done in secrete -under the carpet. Therefore, eradication of sugar relationship among the African Australians remains a mystery to many members of the communities.

The reality is that there are discussions among the African Australians done underground which suggest that there is a growing practice of sugar daddy and sugar baby relationships in the communities — especially between some single fathers (men) and single mothers, as well as between some widows, widowers and other men. It has become abundantly clear that some of the single mothers, widows and housewives are selling their bodies to help meet their family needs, although no one want to talk about it.

The practice of selling bodies appears to be international, although it has not yet been documented in United States of America, Canada, United Kingdom and Europe. It appears that approximately 50% of single mothers, 30% of widows and 15% of housewives from the African community are supporting their lives through undercover sex work (although for the housewives this could be called additional financial support). The research reveals that more and more single mothers, widows and housewives are selling themselves and more African men are buying sex. The study identified that sex sales among the African women are driven by lack of financial resources, which means what the women get from paid jobs or Centrelink is not enough to meet their wants, and this prompts them to engage in sex sales on an ongoing basis. Sarah Daly (2017) observes that although involvement in a sugar baby is typically perceived as deviant and outside the realm of mainstream society, there have been significant changes in the economic, social and cultural acceptance of sexual consumption in the urban economies of Western countries during late capitalism. Females are living in a "sexed-up" culture that has created a more relaxed and liberal attitude towards sex work, thus making the choice to participate in the industry more feasible.

All the African Australian sugar babies participate in indirect sex work, that is why many people think that when African women indirectly sell sex to men this is not considered as prostitution. Development of a sexual relationship usually occurs whenever the woman is enthusiastic about the sex act and makes the man feel special, as though they were in a "consensual non-commercial relationship". Such an experience often involve *hack*, kisses and eventually leads to the sexual act. In addition, the luring of a man may involve going to social gatherings such as a wedding, movies and this may be followed by sexual intercourse in an agreed place. According to Sarah Daly (2017), some scholars argue that the growing demand for sex sellers, who perform feelings of romantic yearning and passion, is part of the "normalization" or "mainstreaming" of sex industries.

What is the meaning of "A Sugar Daddy"?

The term "sugar daddy" may mean differently to different people. However, in this book we are going to adopt the definition of a sugar daddy taken from Dictionary.com, which defines it as "A wealthy, usually older man who gives expensive gifts to a young woman in return for sexual favours or companionship". According to Mia Deboto (2018), sugar dating is a consensual relationship between a financially successful man known as the sugar daddy or brother/uncle, and a female that he financially supports, and that female become known as a "sugar baby".

And what is a sugar baby? Many of us are wondering what the term sugar baby really means and what they do. A sugar baby can be defined as "a person who agrees to be in a transactional relationship for a particular purpose, in general, to achieve financial security. The person is usually attractive, sexy and has a strong sexual appeal. A sugar baby is often misunderstood, and many find it difficult to differentiate it from a prostitute and some people still think it is a prostitute 'under the carpet'.

The research I have conducted, revealed that African Australians define the term "sugar daddy" differently, and from their prospective, a sugar daddy is defined as, "A working man with reasonable income per annum, who could be lured into the practice by some hunting single mothers, widows, as well as some good-for-nothing housewives".

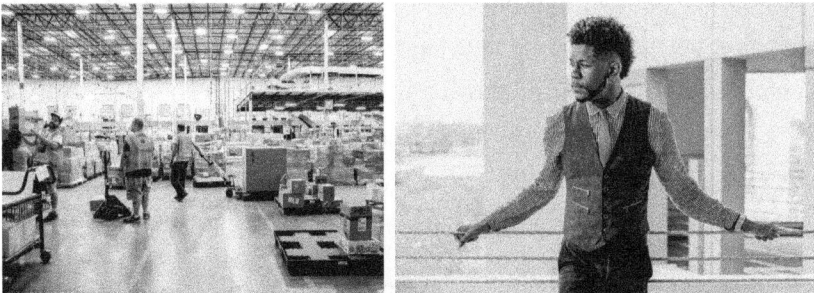

Figure: 11. A Sugar Daddy must be working person

As we have discussed in Chapter 2, African sugar daddies and sugar babies have purposely changed the term "sugar daddy" to "brother or uncle" and they have changed the term "sugar baby" to "sister". The changes of terms have been done for a reason, they want to cover the common terms known globally as "sugar daddy" and "sugar baby" with new disguises, although the terms (brother/uncle and sister) still mean the same. Thus, when the terms are used in this context, foreigners would not understand the meaning behind the terminologies. Subsequently, it becomes difficult for foreigners to know who is "a true brother" or "a true uncle" or "a true sister" to the one calling them so. And this is exactly what the users of sugar relationships want to address.

However, experiences show us that a single mother never uses the term "uncle" or "brother" when introducing a sugar daddy to a relative or a close neighbour. The new terms are usually used when a sugar daddy pays a visit to the house. She does this to throw doubts to friends, children and sometimes a husband, to purposely cover up that a sugar relationship exists between her and the man or a visitor. It is common that African sugar daddies visit their sugar babies in their houses at the weekends. For single mothers, this does not create any problems, but for a housewife who has become a sugar baby this creates problems, because some of the husbands stay at home during weekends. Thus, when a sugar daddy comes into a home of a housewife who has become a sugar baby, and he finds a husband siting in the living room, the usage of the new terminology becomes a problem at this time. The same applies when the man finds the brother of the husband or close relative of the woman in the house. So when this happens, then the term "uncle" is the only appropriate term to be used at this critical time.

So, when a man enters the house, the woman would ask the children (if she has any), "Go and greet your *uncle*". Because the children do not know the man, they will simply trust their mother and greet the visitor as "uncle". The children would each greet the man saying, "Hi uncle, good day or good evening" —depending on the time of the day. The man would also pretend to be a true uncle, telling them, "Oh, children of my sister, I am pleased to see you. I was just passing by. I thought I would come and greet you before going on my way".

Can you imagine what would happen if the husband of the wife was there in the room? When the wife asked the children to go and greet the visitor with the title "uncle", the blood of the husband would run cold.

In African traditional custom, the husband is supposed to know all the brothers, cousins, and close relatives of his wife, and people who usually visit are friends, brothers, sisters, parents or close relatives. So, when a visitor enters the house and a wife asks her children to call a stranger as "uncle", the husband would immediately know that the wife was trying to show him her boyfriend or sugar daddy. Subsequently, the husband has to choose between fighting the man or swallowing a bitter pill. In most cases the man accepts the situation for the sake of the children, but this does not mean that he has forgotten what has happened. When the visitor leaves, the man would ask his wife, "Who was that man?" For majority of women who have become sugar babies, they would not care and just tell the man to his face, "What do you want? Why do you want to know more about him?" This could soon lead to family violence, that might likely be followed by divorce.

This may prompt us to ask a question, "Why do women attract men into sugar relationships? There are many reasons why African single mothers, widows and some housewives attract African males into such unbelievable practices. I have mentioned before that the work of sugar daddy and sugar baby among Africans, is not something new; sugar relationships are not a new phenomenon in the Africa continent. This could be caused by something in the blood or something acquired.

When we look at South Africa, the financial support for single mothers in exchange for sex could go back probably to over 150 years. This was the time when people migrated to the mines and miners (workers) could go home only twice a year; they then went seeking sex around the mines and young girls and some women filled the vacuum.

A study in Kenya by the Communication Company (2002) reveals that two out of three respondents have no problem if someone has a secret wealthy lover. And in Tanzania, previous research showed that most of both young women and their parents find transactional sex acceptable. The relation-ship between a young woman and an old man is called "transactional sex" or "generational sex".

Culturally, in Africa a sugar daddy and sugar baby are not acceptable, but the people are influenced by western ideology especially those whites who come and live together with the people in the new country. Chibwinja Francis (2005), a man from Zambia says," Having a sugar daddy is abominable in the African culture and tradition." (BBC News, 2005). An African man called Leonel Muchano (2005), took the argument further when he said, "Sugar daddies simply dehydrate the moral values of our societies. Rich men make endless offers and promises to young girls; however, if by any chance they find out that their daughters are also going out with a sugar daddy they punish them severely, sometimes unto death".

Having said this, let us come back to Australia where there are many reasons why some African single mothers, widows and some housewives attract African males to be sugar daddies. The women are forced to do this because of the following reasons — divorce, family violence, family break-down, greediness for money, abandonment, death, breakdown of family cultures and structures, the way males and females look at life today, finan-cial control, emotional and physical abuses and the list could go on and on.

What does the word "a single mother" mean?

Some of us struggle to define the words "single mother". There is no general accepted definition of single mother, because different people have differ-ent perceptions of the term. Some dictionaries define "a single mother" as "a mother or woman who does not have a husband or partner". But some writers define it as, "a person who has separated from her husband or partner through legal or illegal divorce or by death of a partner".

However, from the African prospective, a single mother is defined as, "a woman who was previously married and has been separated from the husband through death or divorce and she is waiting for inheritance or remarriage".

Death is beyond the scope of any human being and we must accept it as it is. From the time a person is born, that person will be heading or marching towards death each second, hour, day, week, month and as years pass. The key word here in the definition of a single mother is the phrase "previously married"; most unmarried mothers — although they have babies outside marriage — find it difficult to call themselves as "single mothers". Because the term "single mother" is a heavily loaded term with lots of social and political connotations. According to Emma Johnson (2019), in the Western World, white women do not want to call themselves "single mothers", this is simply to avoid the social stigma that was attached to the term which meant "poor white woman".

It is interesting that the Africans generally do not consider a woman who is legally separated from her husband to be a single mother. They think like this because in Africa cultures, separation and divorce are not acceptable. Africans believe beyond reasonable doubt that "mistakes are made by the man and can be solved by man" — nobody is an angel under the sun.

However, sometimes a widow is called "a single mother", with a loose meaning of the term, to allow her to restructure her life with a potential husband or sugar daddy if she wishes to do so.

Experiences show that single mothers with or without children, have the sole responsibility of providing for herself and children (where applicable). The money received by a single mother from the Australian Government (Centrelink) is just enough for basic needs, but does not cater for increasing daily wants of the people. This is where it becomes necessary for a single mother to look for additional income from a sugar daddy (brother or uncle). Therefore, we can perhaps say that becoming a sugar baby is a necessity and not a choice.

The income of a widow is another thing. The International Committee of the Red Cross and Australian Red Cross found in their workshop held in 1999, that widowhood often changes the social and economic roles of a woman in the household and community, besides altering the structure of the family; its impact differs according to culture and religion. Moreover, widowhood can affect the physical safety, identity and mobility of women and children. It can also affect their access to basic goods and services necessary for survival and their rights to inheritance, land and property, in addition to the wider impact it has on the community.

Why do some married women want to call themselves single mothers?

From daily experiences, we have learned that some women, when their husbands go on a trip for a weekend or have gone overseas for some days, they prefer to call themselves "single mothers". This make us ask ourselves, "What is the motive behind married women calling themselves "single mothers"? Some of the reasons for this may be that the husband often does not give enough money or he hardly does anything around the house; for example, when he is asked to load clothes into washing machines, or when he is asked to unload the dishwasher, he often refuse to do such domestic work. The other reason may be that when women ask their husbands to clean the house, they may refuse. Other reason that some married women may call themselves "single mothers could be that during the night when they want to have sex, the husbands may not want. Eventually, some husbands would never come near their wives for weeks or even months. Therefore, when a woman accumulates all these reasons, it amounts to having no husband.

The worse scenarios are when the women tell their husbands right on their faces that they are not happy with the marriage. Such women forget that every family has problems, and they fail to bring such problems in light -these problems are not openly talked of. Unfortunately, this kind of women, continue discussing family problems with some people who may not even be appropriate to discuss such problems. As a result, such women take family issues onto the streets, and to private places, and keep on telling everyone, especially men saying, "My husband does not give me money, he is not around the house most of the time; I am not happy with our marriage. I am doing everything in the home. I have no husband. I am a single mother". This kind of narrative from the African point of view opens door for a man to whisper in the ears of such hungry women hunting and luring men.

So, when a man hears from a woman that she is a single mother, this can motivate him to approach her. Before long, a man would start to whisper words of love into the ears of a woman. Since the woman is looking for a man, she can accept a man's wishful words. The man then becomes a sugar daddy. However, sometimes such a woman may have a husband and she can become a sugar baby while continuing living with the husband. In most cases, such kind of woman may eventually decide to divorce her husband and become a free woman and continue with sugar relationship. But experiences tell us that when a woman speaks well of her husband, no man will attempt to attract her or to talk to her; every man would fear to approach her.

Although some women go around spreading news that their husbands do not provide money for the family budget, most Africans rebuke this statement because they know that most husbands support their family financially and morally. Even though these husbands support their families, but wives hardly acknowledge such kind of support for the reasons best known to them. Such women are common in African communities in diaspora. Some of them even went as far as claiming they are responsible for everything in the house.

Methods African single mothers use for dating in Australia

It is not easy for a single mother to find a sugar daddy — but they can be found. For the success of the project, a single mother must develop good communication skills and identify possible places where she can find a man of her interest. When a woman meets the man, they would like always to try and know each other. This is important, because if they are going to enter a sugar relationship, they need to know each other more in depth. Before a potential sugar daddy accepts the woman's application, it is important for the man to know what are the basic needs affecting the life of that woman looking for relationship. While the man is identifying the basic needs of the woman, the woman on the other side would be trying to find out if the man is really genuine, honest and willing to pay for any financial assistance she may want — since this relationship is based primarily on money and sex.

During their conversations, at different times and places, there will be lots of questions and answers from each party. Psychologically, a potential sugar daddy would understand the woman from the way she answers questions, he will understand where she is coming from and what exactly she means by saying what she is saying. And by listening to the woman's answers, the man would automatically be arranging the needs of the woman in his mind, where he will categorise them into long-term and short-term needs. At this juncture, it is important to understand that the needs we are talking about here, are more related potential sugar baby and the needs have no connection to the man; because in sugar relationships, men usually do not have needs, but they have wants.

The feelings of the single mother sometimes may become so chaotic and out of control, which often makes her wonder how she will continue for another day.

> *"The relentlessness of single parenthood is draining. You cannot afford to develop a major health problem because no one else is around to take care of your kids. You can't afford to lose your job, or segue to part-time work, because no one else will pay your rent."* By Pauline Gaines (2014)

Histories tell us that single mothers have many needs, but they rarely discuss them with anyone, although some of them tend to discuss the matter with their sisters and friends -if they have one. Some of the single mothers are more like a marble statue, than real persons. And this makes it hard for anyone to connect with them emotionally. For a man to be attracted to a woman he wants, he must first know what her needs are. It is not difficult for a man to find the needs of a woman, it is observed that during conversations, women would normally disclose the undermentioned needs to their potential sugar daddies, and these needs provide the basis on which a man can decide whether to accept the woman as a lover or to reject her. These needs, which are expresses by a woman, may include but are not limited to:

Money: A woman can say, I want a man with money to help address my worries. Money is one of my needs, small things like dry cleaning needs money. So, for our relationship to work well, you must have money to spend".

Material needs: She can also say, "My double bed and mattress are too old in addition I lack modern chairs in my living room; one leg of the dining table is broken and I would like to replace it; my carpets are old and my car is also old it keeps on stopping on the road from time to time.

Children's needs: A woman may say, "My ex-husband does not give enough child support, as a result, when schools open, I find it difficult to buy uniforms, shoes, school bags, books and lunch boxes for my children. For the love of my children, I sometimes decide to go without breakfast and supper to save money primarily for buying school items".

I do not want to fail: A woman may also say, "I want to assure the safety and well-being of my children and myself. I don't want to fail. If something goes wrong in my family, I want somebody who can take or share responsibility".

Feeling constantly guilty: She may say, "I often feel guilty for not seeing my friends and family members as I want to. I also feel guilty for rushing from my place of work to pick children up from school. I also feel guilty that most of the times things are not going according to plan".

Meet people: A woman may say, "I want to meet good matching people in terms of personality, interests and values. I believe this mature match plays a huge part in building strong relationships in my life".

Companionship: A woman may say, "I want to enjoy the best life can offer, but I do not know how I can find this".

Dating someone: She may say, "I am tired of being a single mother. I miss companionship; therefore, I want to go out for dating. Although I can handle my business, I still need someone who is considerate of my situation. I want a person who respects me, love me, and treats me like a smart, beautiful, and intelligent woman in a community. I want someone who has genuine and mature relationship; I want someone with solid friendship that is based on loyalty, and financial support".

Mentorship: A woman may say, " I am looking for somebody that nurtures, guides and genuinely cares about my growth in all aspects of life". Of course, every good teacher needs a good student. This can offer her an opportunity to learn and grow.

Be there for others: A woman may say, "I usually feel lonely; I do not have someone to talk to and to support me. I understand a central pillar of strong relationships is support. I want somebody whom we can connect with and can rely on each other for support when need be."

Connection: She can say, "I want a mentor that can connect me with others outside our world to easily achieve my aspirations".

Be a better me: A woman can say, "I want a better man who can help fulfil my dreams — a good and genuine sugar daddy who can empower and fulfil my life".

I want good night sleeps: A woman may say, "I keep looking on Facebook and YouTube until late at night. My head is often held high to watch and listen for danger that may come at night. I keep one ear open (poised) in case the school calls. I want somebody who can help me go to sleep early so that I have good sleep".

Talking about things that matter to us: She may say, "I want somebody who can talk about real things that matter in our life. I need deep conversation with someone I love". A relationship becomes stronger when a man and a woman discover they believe in the same things and have similar interests. It is these commonalities regarding values and interests that create the strongest emotional connection.

New Experiences: A woman may say, "Life is all about experiences, and experiences come from stepping out of my comfort zone and going for what my heart wants. I want a person with whom we can share our wants and needs. I want to share what I have learned in my life with someone. I feel vulnerable because I keep everything to myself. I want to get out there with somebody to experience the life I always dream about".

Working to bring down stigma: She may say, "I am aware of how my community views me and my children; and above all the way society treats me. Therefore, I want to work hard so that stigma does not pull me down. For this, I need moral support from someone".

Therefore, once a man determines the woman's needs and he has seen her attraction visible, he will then assess on whether to pursue with an official contract or not. Once a man decides to go down the path of a sugar relationship, the next thing he would examine is what a sugar baby will create in their lives. By so doing, a sugar daddy will be finding out what kinds of activities could keep them together, to enjoy life when together. At the same time, a potential sugar daddy makes sure that the woman does not focus too much on his pocket and family members (where applicable).

The period between knowing one another and becoming partners is challenging; during this time, a man and a woman may be exchanging messages to begin getting acquainted with each other. They could exchange messages between 3 — 4 times a day.

Culturally, it is not easy to start speaking about love or a sugar relationship, because African cultures put many restrictions on how the opposite sex could communicate with the other party. However, when a person is driven by the idea of becoming a sugar daddy, he uses all means to get the woman, including modern technology as we have just discussed above. The reality is that, today, the majority of African Australians arrange their sugar relationships over a mobile phone by sending text messages, SMS, photos and sometimes they even chat online.

The modern technology makes it easier for a man to communicate with a woman who lives a distance within minutes. Similarly, a woman can also meet a man in this way. This is good, but unfortunately, they may not know their true characters. It is not enough to see the face of a man or woman in the photos; it is advisable that a person in love must see a picture of the whole body of the person she/he is interested in. Because a man or a woman, in receipt of the picture, cannot determine whether a person in a picture has disability or not. Experience tells us that distance courtship sometimes results in dating a person one does not like.

In the old days, people thought the world was too big as such the communication with other people on the other side of the planet was difficult. But today, the world has become so small that modern technology makes communication easy and accessible. The modern technology also crushes former cultural restrictions as one can reach a person directly and with not much interference (should there be any). Therefore, it is a privilege that, in this modern world, many men and women are dating without much difficulty.

It is reported that dating among African Australians takes between three to eight months, but when we go back to Africa, dating usually takes between one to six years.

However, we should not only stick in saying that some housewives become sugar babies, but it is also reported that some married men are becoming sugar daddies. These men take care of their family members' life as well as sugar baby's life. The sugar babies who befriend married men found it difficult to go out with their sugar daddy during the day but is it usually easier for them to sneak out on the weekend, away from the eyes of the people who may know them. Similarly, housewives who befriend other men found it difficult to go out with them during the day but they easily sneak out on the weekends, and away from the eyes of the people who may know them.

Sugar relationships are top secret

Once the man and the woman are in a sugar relationship, they keep their relationship secret from relatives and friends. Thus, both men and women avoid showing their love in places such as churches and funeral homes for the fear that other people may realise their intentions. It appears that once a man and a woman have come in close sugar relations, before long, they would arrange for meeting in a secret place and none of them would tell the friends these secrete meeting place.

Research found that once a sugar daddy and sugar baby are in love, a sugar daddy would select a day, date, time and place where they would meet. They find it easier to sneak out on the weekend, especially when the husbands are busy with other interests. The housewives also prefer to go out with their men to places where there are no people who may know them. It appears that single mothers and married women find it more convenient to have sex with single men in their houses, as single men live alone in Australia. But if the house of the man or woman is not suitable for meeting, they would prefer to go to a friend's house or to a motel.

It is reported that in the first meeting, after a man and a woman finish their business, a sugar baby would tell a sugar daddy, "I have accepted you to be my man and therefore we have met today. But I don't want you to disclose our sugar relationship to your friends or any member of community. And whenever we meet in public places or in any social gathering, you must pretend as though you do not know me. I will also pretend as though I do not know you. In this way our relationship will remain secret and strong". The man answers, "I will follow your instructions".

"I love you and I am happy that our relationship has not been known by our community and Australian people in general. My idea of this relationship is to help ourselves, you can help me with what you think I need. I can help you sexually any time we have agree to meet. By keeping our relationship secrete because I also want to protect you from community as well as from your family members. For this reason, we cannot go further than this in the country". Source: Rose Mary (2020)

But some sugar babies have no shame whatsoever, and they don't care whether people know about their sugar relationships or not. One woman who had multi-relationships was saying, "Of course, I want to sleep with them; of course, I lie naked in front of them like any normal relationship". In addition, another woman says, "We know it is bad to have multi-relationships, but it is not like we are damaging our reputations; it is just for money".

It is also said that at the first meeting, a sugar daddy or a sugar baby would surprise other with gifts. The person who receives the first gifts would also prepare gifts for the other party. It is generally reported that a person giving the second gift may deliver it on the second or third meetings or even much later. However, there is no timeframe for exchanging gifts. The gifts are usually to demonstrate to each other the generosity. Many of my informants said that such gifts can come in different forms, which may include but not limited to cash of $100 — $500 or above, shoes, camera, handkerchiefs, perfumes, dresses, shirts, handbag, new mobile, etc.

During meetings, some African sugar daddies may even offer to pay at least half of a sugar baby's rent or bills.

May Australians say that some Africans, especially women, are very vocal although some may be closed to themselves. This implies that although some men and women try hard to keep their sugar relationships secret, yet at the end of the day, people will come to know; but nobody will talk about it. The question men and women often fail to answer is, "How long shall we keep our relationship secret?"

Nevertheless, I have been told that some men and women are good at keeping their sugar relationships secret from relatives and friends; subsequently some of them can stay together for 10 years or more without anybody knowing about their relationships. These groups of men and women avoid coming together, especially in places where , communities and friends are meeting.

Differences between African and Anglo-Australian sugar relationships

Having examined the methods of dating and secrecy of sugar relationships among the African Australians, let us now see what the main differences between an African Australian sugar daddy and an Anglo-Australian sugar daddy are. In my research, I have found that there are four main differences and these are:

- ► Firstly, an African sugar daddy exchanges gifts between him and his sugar baby, but an Anglo-Australian sugar daddy does not.

▶ Secondly, an Anglo-Australian man arranges an agreement between him and his sugar baby before supporting her financially, but an African sugar daddy does not.

▶ Third, an Anglo-Australian sugar daddy travels locally and sometimes overseas with his sugar baby, but an African sugar daddy never travels with his sugar baby for the fear that he would expose their relationship to African communities. The man and his sugar baby fear that once they are spotted, they would be challenged publicly. Moreover, some African sugar daddies and sugar babies are said to be dedicated members of some churches and have specific duties within the churches. They fear that if they are seen by members of the church, they would be reported to church authorities and they may be ex-communicated from the respective church.

And for a woman who has befriended a married man, she fears that if the wife (or wives) of the man knew, they would be cursed and rebuked, and sometimes this may lead to fights and divorce. If this happened, it would be considered a disgrace to an African sugar baby. Therefore, this is one of the most important reasons why the African Australian sugar daddies and sugar babies keep their sugar relationships top secret. One of my informants told me that he is involved in a sugar relationship, but this is a secret between him, the woman and God.

But when you look at Anglo-Australians, they have no fear about being known as being in a sugar relationship, because to them this arrangement is legal and accepted by the government — although I have not seen a document showing that the Australian government has accepted this as legal in this country. For the African Australians, although they hear and may have read that the Australian Government regards the work of a sugar daddy and sugar baby as legal, still for them the act is unacceptable. Those Africans who are involved in this are still disturbed by this.

▶ Fourth, an Anglo-Australian sugar daddy pays school fees and rent for his sugar baby, but an African sugar daddy never does this.

Major flirting techniques for women

A sugar baby can never slack off if she wants the relationship to last; the only important thing for the man to do is to be the best-looking and most pleasant self always. The goal is to be a top-notch companion. Moore (1985) observes that verbal communication by a woman to a man she is interested in, does not work in public places such as bars, community gatherings or at English Language Schools, only nonverbal solicitation signals or body movement work better and faster, usually in about 15 minutes. I quite agree with Moore and feel oblige to quote Jeremy Nicholson, M. S. W. PhD (2017) about nonverbal behaviours women use to signal the men they are interested in. According to Jeremy, these nonverbal behaviours include: -

- ▸ Solitary Dance: While seated or standing, the woman moves her body in time to the music playing to draw the man's attention.
- ▸ Room-Encompassing Glance: The woman can look around the room for about 5-10 seconds without making eye contact with others.
- ▸ Short darting Glance: The woman looks at the man of interest sideways for between 2-3 seconds, and when a man recognises the look, he feels a "wave of electric love" running through his blood.
- ▸ Gaze Fixation: The woman makes eye contact with a man of interest for more than 3 seconds.
- ▸ Head Toss: The woman flips her head backwards and lifts her face up briefly. The purpose of this is to attract man's attention.
- ▸ Hair Flip: The woman raises one hand up, touching or pushing it through her hair. This happen only with women with long hair or women who are wearing wigs.
- ▸ Smile: The woman turns the corners of her mouth upward sometimes showing teeth or not.
- ▸ Lean, The woman moves her face and upper body forward, closer to the man. This body language makes a man react positively.
- ▸ Laugh/Giggle: Generally, a woman does this as a response to conversation with a man, at the time they were talking.

▶ Head Nod: Usually while in conversation with a man, she nods in agreement.

When a man has seen one or more of the above behaviours in a woman, he then approaches her, at this time she may be ready to allow her body to be touched by the man in a number of ways; she accepts her body to be touched by the man because she wants to show to him that she is interesting in him. In some cases, a woman may also position herself on the knee of the man, if they are sitting around the same table, so that her knee, thigh or feet touches the man to show interest.

When Moore and Butter (1989) was doing his research, his team were observing the differences in behaviour between single mothers who were approached by men and women who were not approached by men. The result of their observations showed some significant behavioural differences. The study revealed that single mothers who were approached by men often smiled at men when they met; they nod at men, leaned towards them or showed neck presentation.

In contrast, the research showed that women who were not approached by men performed none of the ten flirting behaviours listed above. But single mothers who were approached by men readily look around the room, flip their hair, toss their head and laugh at the glance of a specific man. Interestingly, the study also discovered that the men approach women not because of their behavioural differences, nor their looks, but the study found that a woman who displays a lot of solicitous behaviours is more likely to be approached by men than those attractive women who do not display these behaviours.

But when we talk about flirting, what do we really mean? Flirting is a negotiation process that follows the first meeting between a man and a woman. Attraction plays a big role in finding someone; it is something that needs continuous application in our minds before we decide. Monica Moore (2017) argues that it does not matter whether an attractive person is in a room or not, but what matters most is body contact. Women who smile and make eye contact with others are more likely to be approached, rather than those who are simply good looking. She concluded that for a man and a woman to fall in love they must be in:-

- ▸ Physical Contact — Once a person has become very interested in the opposite sex, she/he shall make body contact by touching a person with hand or leg.

- ▸ Demonstration of traditional flirts — In most human cultures, it is believed that men should make the first move for a relationship; but in other cultures, women may also be allowed to make the first move. In the case where a man is allowed to make the first move, he is expected to take the lead by showing the woman that he is interested in her.

- ▸ Sincere Flirts — As I have mentioned under demonstration of traditional flirts, culturally a man starts flirting to show to the woman that he is sincere and open. By doing this, the man expects a woman to open her heart to him.

- ▸ A study conducted in University of Pennsylvania (2014) revealed that flirters who adjust how overtly they flirt, will have the best success. Some researchers found that flirting has less to do with words or body language, but is more to do with biology. Scientists have long ago speculated on how pheromones or chemicals released into our blood system can have an impact on our contribution to physical attraction. According to Khan Ali (2016) older women are attracted to younger men for a purely biological reason; they know the young men enable them to reach their "prime sexual peak" perfectively well. On the other side, older women are not attracted to older men because they know that older men lose their sexual peak quickly and that would make them angry. Based on this finding, some of the older African women prefer to go after younger men who are ready "to rock their world". It has been said, "No matter how a woman looks, from when she was young up to between 70 or 80 years, she may look very old in the eyes of some men, but the reality is that she is exactly the same person. She has all those impulses and desires for physical touch, for sex, for companionship

— they're still there in her life". In other words, women aged 70-80 are not too old for sex, they are ready for sex with any man they desire.

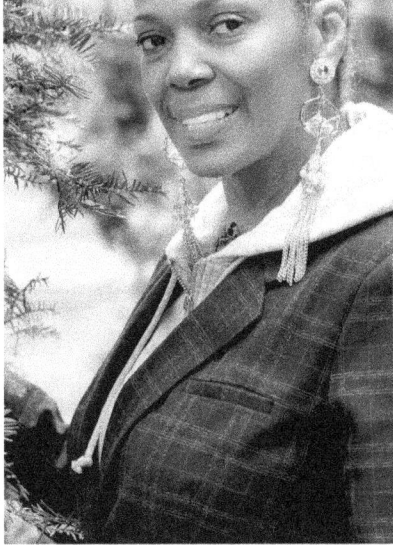

Figure: 13. An older woman who needs a younger man to rock her world.

▶ Gray Miller (2016) took a step further about older women and the sexual act by saying, "Older women prefer having sex with young men not because they are "hot", but there are a lot of other factors that play into the phenomenon". Today, the roles of women have changed dramatically especially in the Western World, where older women are more likely to flirt with younger men, while in Africa older women don't have a choice but they are more interested in any man — regardless whether he is young or matured. For this reason, the older women have acquired their nickname known as "cougars", which means an older woman who hangs out at bars or any public place, looking for any available and willing young men for sex.

▶ In the old days in Australia, an older woman was expected to age gracefully and alone, if she was not married. But today, more Anglo-Australian women are exploring their power and freedom by going back out into the dating scene and finding attractive young men. And these kinds of relationships are not designed to be a long-term or to start a family, it is purely for sexual enjoyment and companionship. I was talking with one of the older Australian women who told me, "I have sexual desire, I can go to have coffee with my boyfriend in his house, and who knows what will happen there?"

▶ Having examined all aspects of older women, we cannot deny that in Australia there are some African older women who are aging gracefully alone and are still sexually active. It is very easy to identify such older and sexually active women in the community. The common indicators are first, she is always smart and keeps herself attractive to men; second, she always flirts with men, especially through love smiles and blinking of the eyes. In contrast, some African older women (of the same age 65-80) do not want to talk or hear about sex. One day, when I went to visit an older African woman during my research and as we were discussing about sugar relationships, she told me, "We old African women have left sexual enjoyment to our daughters and other young women. Our time has gone. I know there are some old African women who are still interested in sexual intercourse, this is not good; it is degrading in society".

What is a sugar mummy?

When I was doing my research about sugar relationships among African Australians, I went to Pakenham library (in Victoria State) with the aim to get books about the topic. To my surprise, a librarian, who happened to be an Anglo-Australian woman, told me that she has never heard about a sugar mummy, but she knows about a sugar daddy and sugar baby. The other female member in the library also told me, "I never knew that sugar mummies existed. I only know that sugar daddies and sugar babies exist. I do not know if sugar mummies even exist in Australia," she said. When I went around other rural libraries in the South Eastern suburbs of Melbourne, I was told categorically, "We have no books about sugar mummy in our libraries. We only know sugar daddies and sugar babies exist; this is the first time we are hearing from you that sugar mummies also exist. And Librarian asked me, "Do sugar mummies really exist in the modern world?" I could not answer this question, as I was still on my fact-finding mission.

I started to ask myself, "What is a sugar mummy and what do they do?" According to ToyBoyDates website, a sugar mummy is defined as "An older woman who spends money on a younger person, usually in exchange for romantic and sexual purposes". Sugar mummies are found across the world although the level of sugar mothers varies from country to country.

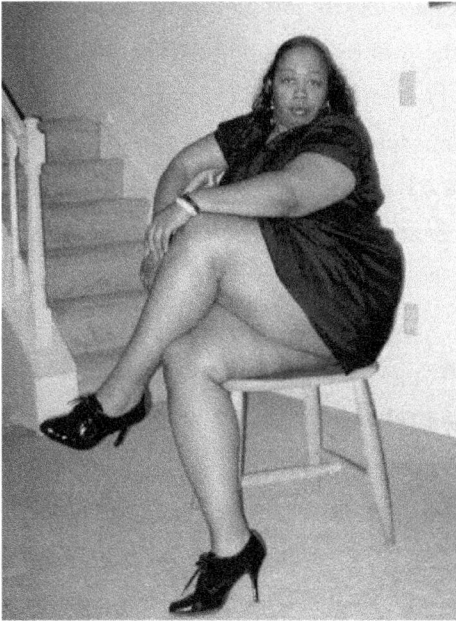

Figure: 12. A Sugar Mother

I went further to ask myself, "What is the difference between a sugar daddy and a sugar mummy? Many writers reported that the difference only lies in gender, a sugar mummy is a female, and a sugar daddy is a male; yet both use money to buy gifts for either a young man or young woman, and to flirt with them for romantic or sexual purposes.

The other difference between a sugar mummy and a sugar daddy is that a sugar daddy does not look for a woman, but it is a woman who looks for him; in contrast, sugar mummy looks for a young man. A sugar mummy tends to use her money as a means to flirt with young men; a sugar mummy usually has less interest in mature men. In different parts of the world some people call a "sugar mummy" as "sugar mother", while in other parts of the world they call them "sugar mommas" or "cougars", these calls depend on where one lives. Sugar mothers support their sugar babies the same way mothers treat their babies.

Some young men in the community want to connect with sugar mothers, but they do not know how to find them. In my research I found that there are no sugar mothers among African Australians; but if someone wants to connect with Anglo sugar mummies, the best place to find them is through online websites/apps specified as a Sugar Arrangement. This is a place where sugar mothers are actively looking for young men; however, don't forget that some sugar mothers do not use their true names, it is up to you to find out. And when you are in conversation with a sugar mother, whether online or over the phone, ask more questions about the subject and if she tells you her true name, repeat it once or twice until you learn it.

One of strange things about a sugar relationship with a sugar mother is that once a man relates to her, that man will be called "sugar baby". Therefore, the term sugar baby does not only apply for a woman, but it also applies to a man. A man will become a sugar baby to a sugar mother and a woman or girl will become a sugar baby to a sugar daddy.

It is estimated that a sugar mummy in the Western World earns $250,000 per annum and she could give as much as $2,800 to her sugar baby (young man) a month.

In Australia, a good number of African women are working. Their main jobs include in age care, disability, child care, hospitality and factories. Their salaries range between $50,000 to $100,000 per annum. Therefore, the income received by African Australian women, does not qualify them to be a sugar mummy. Research revealed that African women living in Australia, they have higher demands and lower income. And some African men living in Australia, somehow, receive higher annual income which qualifies them to be sugar daddies.

Flirting is important in the life of a person who wants to be a sugar daddy or sugar mother, and study shows that there are many reasons why some men and some women want to flirt in the human society. Here are three top reasons why men and sugar mothers want to flirt:

- Sex — the "flirter" usually wants to get into bed with the person she/ he is attracted to.
- Fun — it is reported that some men and women regard flirtation as a sport.
- Trying to find a companion — It is observed that men and women whisper in the ears of a partner because they are searching for intimacy.

How do men perceive women's sexual interest?

When I talk of "men" in this context, I mean all men whether they are white, black, yellow, light skin or brown, and regardless where they come from. Men's perceptions of women's sexual interest were studied in a sample of 250 males, which revealed that these men differed in their thinking about women sexual interest base on attractiveness, provocativeness of dress, and the social environment. Study found that men's judgements about women's sexual interest have been influenced by their own environment. But in reality, women sexual interests are dependent personal sexual interest and how they are been provoke and how attractive they appear in the society. Analysis of individual differences in cue usage suggested that men's judgement about women's momentary sexual interest varied along two dimensions: firstly, there were men who relied on affective cues and they were less likely to response to women's attractiveness; the second group of men were those men who were influenced more by provocativeness of dress women worn, and this group were more relying on the environmental context in their judgements. It was found that men who have misconception about sexual interest in their wives often develop aggressive behaviour. As a result, the study suggested that variation in contextual variables should be included in cognitive-training programs designed to improve the accuracy of men's judgements of women's responses. (Teresa A. Treat et al. 2016).

Male-initiated sexual aggression toward female acquaintances is a serious behavioural health problem across human societies. Current theories suggest that misperception of the sexual interest of a potential partner, may increase the likelihood of sexually coercive and aggressive behaviour. The emotional cues that a woman expresses on her face and with her body provide a clear nonverbal indicator, which show how she feels about a man at a particular point in time. As we have seen from the arguments of Teresa A. Treat (2016) above, when judging sexual interest in women, men focus not only on emotional cues, but they also focus on the provocativeness of women's clothing and their attractiveness. Surprisingly, when judging women's current sexual interest men rely heavily on women's nonverbal actions.

It appears that among heterosexual people, men tend to over-perceive sexual interest in women, while women tend to under-perceive sexual interest in men. Thus, it is very common and difficult to perceive someone's level of sexual interest at any point of time. However, a man's misperception about woman's level of sexual interest are usually minor but yet we can say it is embarrassing social error. This means the man may assume that a woman could be more sexually interested than she really is or he may assume that a woman is less more interested in sex than she actually is. Teresa A. Treat et al (2016) observes, "Men's misperception of a female partner's sexual interest is not only a normative phenomenon affecting most men, but also a potentially clinically relevant phenomenon. Misperception is associated both theoretically and empirically among men with an increased risk of exhibiting sexually coercive and aggressive behaviour toward acquaintances, as commonly indicated by endorsement of rape-supportive attitudes."

The general findings of the study are summarised under four psychological sub-headings: sexual interest utilization effects; Provocativeness of dress utilization effects; Attractiveness utilization effects and Sexual relevance utilization effects. So, when men are judging women's sexual interest, they rely on these four psychological dimensions. Let us now examine these four dimensions one by one.

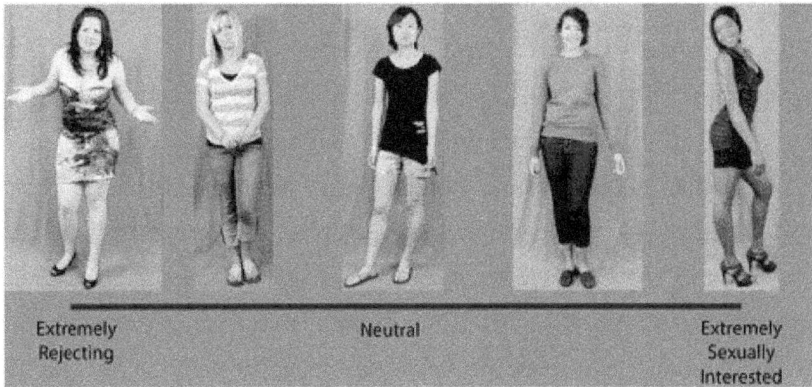

| Extremely Rejecting | Neutral | Extremely Sexually Interested |

Figure 13: Men's Judgement of Women

The 250 males were to give their perceptions about sexual interest in the five women who were taken in their full-body photos. They have divided the women into three groups, where one group was wearing full-body dress and were expressing their inner sexual interest. The second group of women were not fully-body dress and the third group of women were wearing short-skirt dress. The four psychological dimensions use to judge women's sexual interest were as follows:

Sexual interest effects: When judging the women, about sexual interest, the participants relied very strongly on how women feel sexually. The group found that rape-supportive attitudes predicted by men reduced reliance on affection. A woman can be raped, and this would not necessarily mean that she is lovely. Thus, the higher-risk men always tend to make is that they focus less on women's affection but rather judge women on the basis that they are ever sexually interested (sexually ready).

Provocativeness of dress and its effects: The group of men, who were working with the second group of women, focused more on women's clothing style, when they were judging their momentary sexual interest. They found that some men are attracted to the dress (the way a woman dress) as a result this group of men can easily rape a woman because of the attitudes they have about clothing style. For example, from Figure 13, women with short skirts or dress are more likely to be raped because men think these women are advertising themselves -they are sexually interested.

Attractiveness: What makes a person sexually attracted to another remains a mystery as no scholar has found an answer to it. There is no standard measure for perceptions of sexual attractiveness. The self-perceived sexual attractiveness (SPSA) scale is now developed. If one is interested in using this scale, he/she can do so. The new scale is a valid and reliable measure of self-perceived sexual attractiveness that may be used among men and women who identify as heterosexual, gay, lesbian or bisexual. The men who were asked to judge the five women in figure 13, they focused their attention more on "attractiveness and its effects". They concluded that attractive women are more likely to be raped than non-attractive women. (I personally don't believe with this group of men, for me all women whether attractive or non-attractive are always sexually interested). They assumed that attractive women are usually sexually interested. And the attractiveness of such women is based on their normal dresses. The study also found that men with aggressive behaviour towards their wives don't focus on them, but they focus more on their wives' characteristics.

Contextual Sexual Relevance: A sexual context is provisionally defined as an environment that tends in most reproductively active to provoke further sexual stimulation or self-stimulation to ejaculate. The men who were assigned to judge sexual interest in those five women, relied moderately on the sexual relevance of the context, that is which environment could let a woman become sexually interested. They found that women can be sexually interested depending on the environment. If the environment is safe for sex, she can be more sexually interested but is the environment is not safe she may have less interest in sex. In other words, she may not be ready for sex.

Therefore, unsafe environment offers low risk for a woman because she may not even want to go there. This means she has low risk for rape.

From our point of view in this book, sexual relevant contexts are associated with dating and sexual activity, but a woman's level of sexual interest within these contexts may fluctuate over time and vary according to the interest she has in a man.

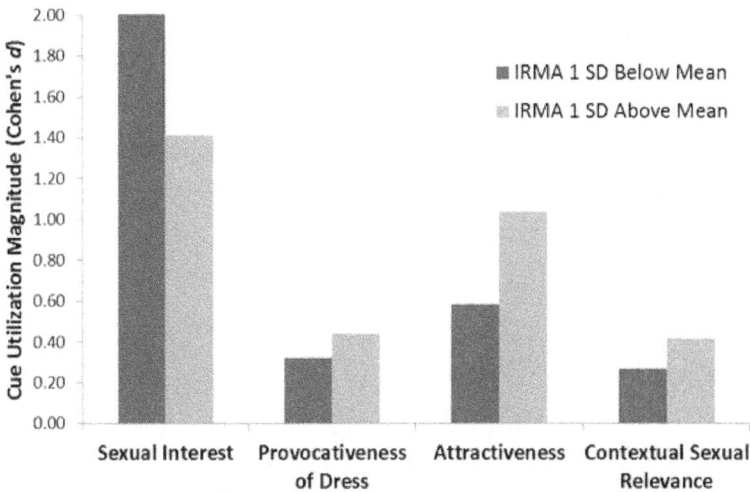

Source: Teresa A. Treat (2016). Men's perception of women's sexual interest

Common places for finding a sugar daddy and sugar baby in Australia

There are many places in Australia, where African men and women can find a person to start sugar relationships. Experiences of African communities show that single mothers, widows and some housewives attract men for dating, by associating it with sex, in the following top ten places:

▸ Churches
▸ Funeral places
▸ Community meetings
▸ Adult Migrant Education Services

- ▸ Technical and Further Education (TAFE)
- ▸ In the workplace
- ▸ Supermarkets
- ▸ In buses
- ▸ In trains and train stations
- ▸ In houses.

I have learned from community conversations that the abovementioned places are the most common places where single mothers, widows and some housewives attract men, and vice versa, these are the places where men, who are looking for sugar babies, hang around. It appears that in these places, aural conversation is not necessary or important, but in these places men and women use body language because body language speaks louder than words.

Chapter Four
Multiple Sugar Daddies

What does it mean to have multiple sugar daddies and sugar babies?

In this book when we talk of having multiple sugar daddies or multiple sugar babies, this is when a man is having sexual relationships with more than one woman or when a woman is having sexual relationships with more than one man. It is reported that in the African Australia community, some men or women have between 2 — 6 sexual relationships with the opposite sex.

But in general, it is said that many African Australians do not like having multiple sugar daddies or sugar babies, but the reality is that some of them do. African Australian women who engage in multiple sugar daddies are driven into the practice by greed for money and they are mainly forced into it because of divorce and separation. While African men who are engaged in multiple sugar babies are driven by their lust and pride of having sex with as many women as possible. Reports coming from the African continent, state that many young girls and young men are now involved in multiple sugar relationships. However, I want to emphasize that multiple sugar relationships can be bad for the health of the women as well as for the health of the men.

It appears that both men and women, who are practising multiple sugar relationships, have failed to understand that having too many sexual relationships has its own consequences. The first consequence that multiple sexual relationships bring to a man is that it drains his income; secondly it exposes him to STDs. And for a woman, multiple sexual sugar relationships firstly expose her to STDs and secondly, may affect a woman's future marriage — if she decides to go down that path.

Having said this, let us look at a true story from Nigeria, written by Faka Oludo in January 2020. Mr Osamudiame Iyobosa was married to Mrs Edeki, and during their dating period they never had sex. This was because they were following the strict African custom that forbids a man and woman to have sexual intercourse before marriage. The story of the couple goes as follows, "After a few days of living together, Mr Iyobosa decided to return his wife to her parents because he discovered that her vagina was too wide. Everybody was in shock at Ebelle community in Edo State.

The community was amused at how the man could be that childish as to return his legally married wife for such a flimsy excuse. When the man dropped his wife at her parents' house in Ubiaja, he told his in-laws that many men must have slept with Edeki, as he found her vagina too wide.

When this news spread around the town, a man who sells palm wine near Ubiaja market admitted that the husband may be right, as according to him, Edeki (the wife) was a well-known flirt in the neighbourhood and that no indigene would have married her. The man said they were surprised when Iyobosa (the husband) came from Benin to marry her. Some young girls even started flirting because they said Edeki was lucky. Whenever these girls are talking about sugar relationships, they usually give Edeki as an example of a lucky flirt.

The parents of Edeki were very angry with their son-in-law for exposing their daughter's weakness publicly. The mother of the girl then called her son-in-law "half man".

Some members of community said this was strange, as no man had ever done this in their community by returning his wife to her parents because she had a too-wide vagina. The worst thing was that Iyobosa told onlookers that his wife had an 'expressway pussy'." Source: shakarasquare.com, 2020.

From the above narrative, we can easily see how multiple sexual relationships can impact on women who may want to get married after previous long sexual and paid relationships.

However, entering the roles of sugar daddies and sugar babies appears very exciting to some of the African men and women. It has been reported that entering the 'sugar bowl' is not easy; it requires self-advertisement. Some women think that by having sugar daddies they have a stress-free lifestyle, since they will be receiving monthly financial support from every sugar daddy. It is assumed that the more sugar daddies have sugar babies, the more monthly allowances each woman would have, and the more ability that woman will have to meet her needs. This is the main reason why some African Australian sugar babies want to have multiple sugar relationships, they do this so that they get as much money as possible out of their time in the "sugar bowl".

A verbal report says that most African Australian sugar babies are doing it right and they get the most out of it. Every sugar baby has her own objectives and lucrative opinions to finance their families, as it offers additional income. So the underground selling of sex has become the best option to get some more funds into the family budget.

One lady was saying, "*I don't care what people think, feel and talk about me. My body belongs to me, I can use my body the way I want. I can sleep with as many men as I want to achieve my goals*".

Below is a true history from a well-known African Australian sugar baby; because of privacy and confidentiality, she wants to be known by the name Rose Mary which is not her real name.

Mrs Mary says, "I am a married woman with eight children; each of the children has different father. They have different fathers because I have multiple sugar daddies. I decided to have multiple sugar daddies because when I married my true husband, after a year and a half, I came to know that my husband was not productive. When we were in bed my husband played sex well and he has normal ejaculation. But after a year of staying together I was not pregnant; I was looking for a child or children. So, we visited a doctor, who told us that although my husband is sexually active, his sperm is weak, and he cannot produce a child. Although my husband has a high political position in the government, his income was low; but I decided not to divorce him. So, I decided to look for some men the first man I met was my college mate and I had a child with him. My primary aim was to have as many children as I can. So, before long, I was pregnant with my second child with another man. When my second child turned one year and a half old, I found another sugar daddy and had my third child. The games went on and on, I kept on moving from one man to another, until I have had my eight children. This explain why each of my child have a different father; It was unfortunate, I never had a long-term sugar relationship with one man, I moved from man to man purely for sexual enjoyment and money."

Sarah Daly (2012) observes that the cost of living in our world today and increased pressure of unmet demands has contributed to women selling sex. Another reason is the lack of employment, which largely comprises casual and part-time, uncertain and low paid jobs. Some single mothers, widows and housewives indicated that the sale of sex is an attractive thing to do. In the area of sugar daddies and sugar babies, it is usually hard to be honest with oneself to have only one sugar daddy (uncle) or sugar baby (sister). Therefore, these women and men who prefer to "double dip", we can say they have stuck their toes into multi-relationships.

However, one thing African Australian sugar babies fail to understand is that having more than one sugar daddy comes with responsibilities, time commitments and the willingness to be honest with oneself and each of the men she is having sex with. It is said that after spending some months with a sugar baby, every one of the men would like to know if she has another man on the side. This question usually challenges the honesty of a woman; history tells us that no African woman would admit to her sugar daddy or a husband that she has another man or two on the side. Although a sugar baby would not admit to her sugar daddy or husband that she has another man on the side, many African men ask such a question because of the following top eight reasons:-

▶ Because the man does not want to share a woman with another man, especially a woman he is supporting financially every month.

▶ Because the man wants to know whether there could be a chance for him to expose himself to sexual transmitted diseases (STDs); this could jeopardize their relationship. It is true that African men generally do not like to use condoms, therefore, if a woman has another man on the side, he will prefer to separate from her. Nancy Luke (2005) observed in the early stages of the HIV/AID epidemic in sub-Saharan Africa, that economic status was positively associated with HIV infections. Although having multiple sugar daddies does have benefits, sexual transmitted diseases don't. As a matter of fact, it is always difficult to know who has STDs and who doesn't.

▶ If a sugar baby is going with other men, a man may find it sexually enticing to think of a sugar baby with other men.

▶ Having more than one man may be difficult for a woman to keep to the different appointments made by each man — eventually some appointments may coincide, and she has to cancel one and go with the other. A man whose appointment is cancelled usually feels angry about this.

▶ When there are lots of appointment cancellations and rescheduling to suit a woman's timetable, this becomes a clear indication that a woman has other men to attend to.

▶ Many women are not happy when a sugar daddy calls her when she is in a room with another sugar daddy. In many cases when this happens, a woman will not pick up her mobile, and when the man she is attending to, asks her to answer the mobile, she could easily say, "I am tired of such calls from overseas". But if by accident she picks up the mobile and a man says, "Hi darling, I love you", she will simply give a short answer, "Me too," instead of saying, "I love you too". She is giving this short answer to confuse the man she is attending to so he would not know that the call is coming from another sugar daddy.

- ▸ Because if a sugar baby has multiple males, she is no longer considered a sugar baby but rather a prostitute.
- ▸ Having many men, a woman can fake her orgasm but she cannot fake how she really feels about someone. Therefore, when a woman begins to smell differently than usual, this means there is another "bull is around the corner".

Female external genitalia

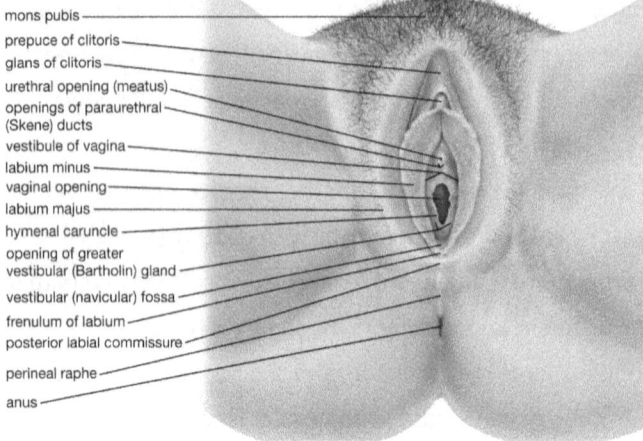

mons pubis
prepuce of clitoris
glans of clitoris
urethral opening (meatus)
openings of paraurethral (Skene) ducts
vestibule of vagina
labium minus
vaginal opening
labium majus
hymenal caruncle
opening of greater vestibular (Bartholin) gland
vestibular (navicular) fossa
frenulum of labium
posterior labial commissure
perineal raphe
anus

Figure: 14. A woman can fake her orgasm

From the eight reasons given above, it could be possible that while the man is having sex with his sugar baby, he could also be having sex with other women who may have STDs, in which case he could pass on the disease to his partner/wife. Similarly, a woman with multiple sugar daddies may contract STDs and spread them to other men, including her husband if she is married. Therefore, this book wants to create awareness to the African Australians to know that there are lots of things in a sugar relationship to be mindful of. If a sugar baby has STDs, she will be in constant fear that her past may be exposed; this same fear applies to a man. Thus, this is a terrible psychological burden that may affect a person for the rest of her/his life.

A sugar baby is never transparent and honest

As I mentioned before, a woman in a sugar relationship will not be transparent, honest and open to her man for the fear that she may lose him, as losing a sugar daddy means losing money, since their relationship is simply based on money.

It is believed that any African man who becomes a sugar daddy, does not want a sugar baby to come to him grumbling with the problems and stresses of her life. Rather, an African man wants a woman who can inject happiness and hope into his life.

As we have discussed above, sugar relationships across the world are based on money. Therefore, African Australian sugar babies are no exception; today it appears the average African Australian sugar baby receives between $300 and $1,500 a month from one man. Some men may give more than what sugar babies expect, because they want to stop their sugar babies from having sexual intercourse with other men. But this appears not to work, as some women who are hungry for money won't consider the offer and still go with other men to boost their financial position.

One of my informants Mr Obalkara, told me that he has been in a sugar relationship with Ms Mpande (not their real names) for nine years. Mr Obalkara said they planned to have sex twice a month, but before long Ms Mpande became reluctant, and as a result it was reduced from 2 to 1 sexual relationship a month in a motel. Mr Obalkara revealed that Ms Mpande wanted more money rather than more sexual services and this led him to drop the relationship after nine years. Mr Obalkara claimed that sex once a month is not worth the $1,000, he spends on Ms Mpande per month. From the above narrative, we can see clearly how sugar babies are never transparent and honest.

Tips for juggling two or more sugar daddies

I have brought this topic here, not because I want to encourage the practice of sugar daddy and sugar baby among the African Australians, but because it appears that there are some women, who would like to practice and continue with multiple relationships.

It is said that most sugar babies start their relationship by having one sugar daddy. After this, she may have man or men. By doing this, a woman may think that she is more likely to have a luxurious lifestyle and have more money in her bank account. Thus, if any African woman outside there wants to enter the business, she should follow these five tips: -

▶ Schedule your time well: In doing this, you need to figure out where you think you can fit time in with your second or third sugar daddy. This time must work for both parties, so that things don't get too complicated.

▶ Let your first sugar daddy be your first priority: As a human being you might tend to favour one man more than the other, but this does not mean you give less attention to either one. You should remember that time is precious to all; each needs to feel important even though they don't know the other men involved.

▶ Keep your phone away when you are having time together with your man: Modern technologies have become a disease for both adults and young people. Some people cannot spend 5 minutes without looking at their phone. So, it is always advisable when you are with your man, to put your phone aside and focus on the person with whom you are in the room. Give him your undivided attention; put his needs first when you are with him. This same rule applies when you are with the other men.

▶ Create a genuine connection with each sugar daddy: It is generally believed that by creating a connection, this will make you want to spend equal time and want to see each of them. And when you are with them, speak the sweetest words you have ever kept in the bottom of your heart. This kind of connection goes back to making them feel important. Your extra time spent on another man will not feel beneficial if you are faking your feelings and it will soon feel like a chore.

▶ Make time for yourself: This is very important because by having multiple sugar daddies, this can easily take up your time for your regular commitments. You need to find time to go out shopping and visiting your friends and family members, to attend community meetings, and time to visit each of the men. Thus, having multiple sugar daddies if you don't manage your time well can make your life unenjoyable.

Tips to being a good sugar daddy (brother or uncle)

I know there are some African Australians who would like to become good sugar daddy or uncle, but they do not know how to become a good sugar daddy. Research reveals that there are eleven top tips that a man could follow to enable him to become a good sugar daddy. Before we examine the eleven steps, I would like to inform men that these steps involve personal commitment. The eleven tips or steps are as follows:-

► Talk to a woman you are interested in (single mother, widow or house-wife): No woman can know that a man is interested in her unless he (the man) communicate his feelings. Culturally, it is a man that starts the game and not a woman. As I have just said above if a man does not talk to a woman, she will never know what is in his heart and mind, therefore communication is very important.

► Find out the basic needs of the woman: Study shows that each woman has her own basic needs which may be different from the needs of other women. When a woman is talking about the needs, the man should understand that there are many types of needs, which include clothes, shoes, money for paying rent or bills, watches, new mobile phones, car services, bed sheets and blankets at winter time, support to relatives overseas and many more.

► Make a proposition on how you can meet her needs: Don't think that when a woman sees a man, she would immediately know that he is the right person for her. This is not true, as many sugar babies want to know whether you are the right sugar daddy, who can help address some of her burning needs, she wants to hear you making some proposals (i.e. what you help her with). As a man, you should know that a woman, who is interested in you, prefers to hear some proposals from you. The common proposals man usually make include saying thing such as, "I am ready to help you financially and will stand by you in whatever situation that may arise".

▸ Don't talk to a woman you are interested in about her past mistakes: This woman may be known to you for some time, but when you are talking to her about your interest, don't talk about her past mistakes (bad actions or some of her misbehaviour you might have known about). If you do this, it can scare her from you and make you a bad sugar daddy. It is generally believed that for a woman to develop a relationship with a man, she wants the man to be ignorant of her past misbehaviours, and more importantly, the man should not know her background — especially her dark side. If a woman understands that you know of her past behaviours and family background, she will not accept you as a lover.

▸ When talking to a woman, be straightforward, don't beat around the bush with matters of importance: Study shows that sugar babies are usually straightforward when dealing with a man; they like telling their needs and what they expect from a man. A good example is, "There was a man who had fallen in love with a single mother and they decided to spend the first night in her house. There, the woman told him to his face, "Now, you want me, so for our love to be strong I want you to build a house for my mother in Africa". The man was not ready for the woman's demand; so he immediately stopped the relationship. This tells us that if this man had much interest in the woman, he would have told her simply, "OK honey, let us give ourselves time and thing will be done". If the man was to answer the woman in this way, this would have given hope to the woman and the relationship would have continue.

▸ Misunderstanding is normal: There is no relationship or marriage under the sun that goes without misunderstanding. When you are interested in a woman, you should understand and expect from day one that misunderstandings may arise in the course of time. For this reason, a man must be ready for forgiveness.

- ▶ Forgiveness is of paramount important in any relationship: As I have just mentioned above, misunderstanding is normal in any relationship and it can happen anytime. So, if you want to be a good sugar daddy, you must find a place in your heart for forgiveness.

- ▶ Avoid a woman who is totally dependent on you: It appears some women want to be totally dependent on a sugar daddy. Thus, if you want to be a good sugar daddy, don't allow a woman that you love to depend entirely on you, because one day if you fail to support her financially, that will be the end of relationship.

- ▶ Indicate your trustfulness to a woman: Most women want to have men who are trusted. So, if you want to be a good man to your sugar baby, show her at all times that you are a good trusted friend. In this case, your relationship will last longer or forever, otherwise your relationship may not last for long as you expected

- ▶ Don't tell lies to your sugar baby: It is common that a man and a woman in love often discuss their affairs. This is perfectly normal, but study shows that when talking about your affairs, avoid telling lies, because once she finds out that you are telling lies, she will abandon you and look for another man.

- ▶ Look your best look all the time: Body image is important for both men and women. Women want to see their partner well dressed all the time. Therefore, be the best looking person and most pleasant always, especially in the places where both of you meet. A woman does not like a man who looks poorly and with a smelly body and mouth. Therefore, have a regular bath and brush your teeth twice a day.

Changing economic and social landscape

Marketing of sex among African Australian women, that was supposed to be a privatized product, is now sold to men underground; and most likely some women might be selling sex alongside mainstream industries. It is believed that African women who want to sell sex in mainstream industries, go a distance from where they live to look for the market. This means that if a woman lives in Moe or Narre Warren, she drives to Melbourne city to sell sex, where she is not known to the people. By the term "mainstream" we refer to the expansion of the sex industries in Australia, where sex workers are accepted and the act is lawful. This is a place where conventional business models are used with increased visibility and a growing number of sex workers. The trend encourages the normalization of the sex industry in women across Australia. According to Sarah Daly (2017), mainstreaming is facilitated through the process of divorce and separations, which involved moving away from a joint income to a single income; and this is also the time when a sugar daddy (uncle) and sugar baby (sister) are made more desirable. As a result, women become unselfconscious about their participation in these relationships, because they think this is the only way forward after divorce or separation. This is the disillusion rather than transformation to independency. (P. 16)

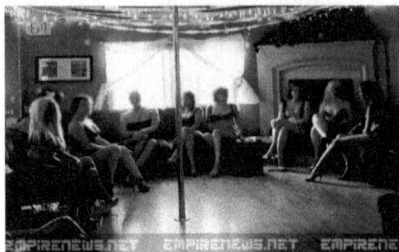

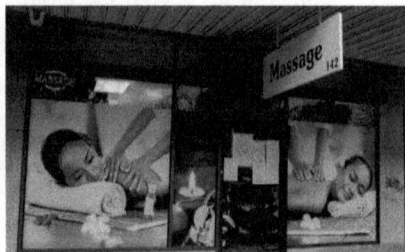

Figure: 15. Sex workers in brothel Figure: 16. Happy Ending Massage centre

Today in Australia, the market has found its root in African Australian women who are divorced or separated. The practices have become common and without shame. For this reason, sexual relationships, among African Australians have been fashioned into commodities, creating a new name for "sugar daddy" to "brother or uncle" and for "sugar baby" to "sister"; the experiences of becoming a "brother" or "sister" is connected with selling and buying sex. Emotional connectedness through mutual satisfaction, love and friendship enables the African Australian sugar baby's experience to be marketed and consumed.

The enhanced meaning of "brother or uncle" and "sister" purchased through underground commercial sex, contributes to new forms of sexual and emotional labour, which provide viable economic earning and power for some women, as well as a desired commodity for some African men to buy fantasies.

Having discussed this, we should not forget that many facets of African Australian communities are influenced by widowhood, and the effects of widowhood have consequences on them. In the Western World, like Australia, widowhood is studied from various perspectives that include remarriage (the study covers demography, economics and a social life of a person). In contrast, the majority of African women who are divorced or become widows have slim chances for remarriage—and the sugar baby has become the job for the day.

Chapter Five
Genital Sores And Rash

Female genital sores and rash

Many women cannot explain what genital sores and rashes are, although they experience it in their vagina. For the sake of those who are interested in knowing the meaning of the sores and rash, here is the explanation of one of the writers Debra Rose Wilson (2019) and she says, "Female genital sores are bumps and blisters in or around the vagina. They may appear as small, red or flesh-coloured bumps and blisters. Some sores may be itchy, painful, and tender or produce a discharge. But others may not cause any symptoms". It often occurs as a result of taking antibiotics. However, there are many conditions that can cause a woman to develop a rash around her vagina; some are minor, and others more serious. Men can also develop a genital rash on the head of their penis, as we can see in the figure 18 below.

However, sores on the genitals sometimes happen for no reason and can resolve on their own; others may be due to certain skin disorders and these may be symptoms of a sexually transmitted infection (STI) and this are normally associated with symptoms such as:-

- Painful intercourse
- Discomfort when urinating
- Increased or foul-smelling vagina discharge.

It is reported that young women are more at risk for developing serious long-term health complications resulting from untreated infections.

A genital rash can cause worry, especially if the reason for it is not fully understood. In most cases, a genital rash is a symptom of another disorder. A genital rash typically refers to a spread of bumps, lesions or irregular patches of skin on the vagina. (Suzanne Falck, 2018).

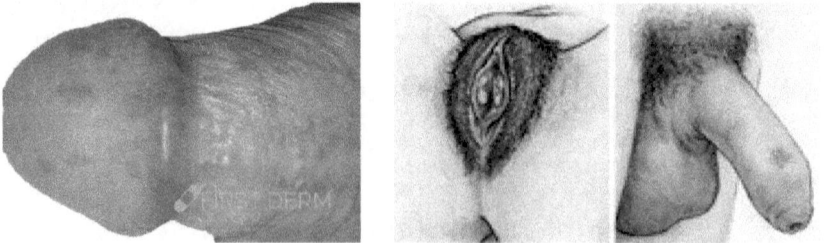

Figure: 17. Genitals rash

Therefore, if a person notices painful swelling around the genital area, she or he should speak to a doctor — it could be a sign of a nasty infection. If this is not treated, it could cause pain and discomfort which a woman or a man may not want.

As I have just explained above, some women may not know what the sores and rash are or its symptoms. So how can a woman recognise that she has a genital sore? It is true genital sores may appear as small, red or flesh-coloured bumps and blisters and it may be difficult for some women to recognise them. More importantly, sores may change appearance and become crusty or larger. Therefore, a woman can recognise that she has genital sore only when it is accompanied by the following symptoms:

- ► Itching at the site
- ► Pelvic pain
- ► Burning
- ► Bleeding
- ► Discomfort when urinating

Similarly, a woman may recognise that she has a genital rash when she can see the following symptoms in her body: —

- ► Sores, bumps, blisters or lesions on the skin, on and around the genitals

- ▶ Thickening of affected skin
- ▶ Irritation or inflammation
- ▶ Itching or burning sensations
- ▶ Discoloured skin ranging from pink, red to yellow
- ▶ Discharge from the genitals
- ▶ Pain during intercourse
- ▶ Pelvic pain
- ▶ Fever
- ▶ Enlarged lymph nodes.

In this modern world, with modern techniques we can avoid rashes caused by STIs when we use safe sex. This means that a man must use condoms, but unfortunately, some African Australian men do not want to use condoms because they think that using condoms is no different to masturbation — they go for sex with a woman because they do not want masturbation.

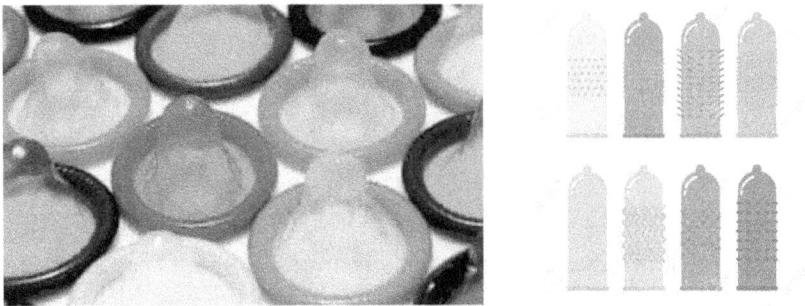

Figure: 18. Condoms for safe sex

Therefore, this means that men who do not use condoms are more likely at risk for genital sores and rashes than those who use condoms. Some men claim that they are allergic to condoms, and the only way to prevent allergic reactions is by avoiding the things that trigger the allergies, such as condoms.

In most cases, sores can be cured with treatment. At this point, it is important to note that sores due to genital herpes or a chronic skin condition may re-occur in a woman.

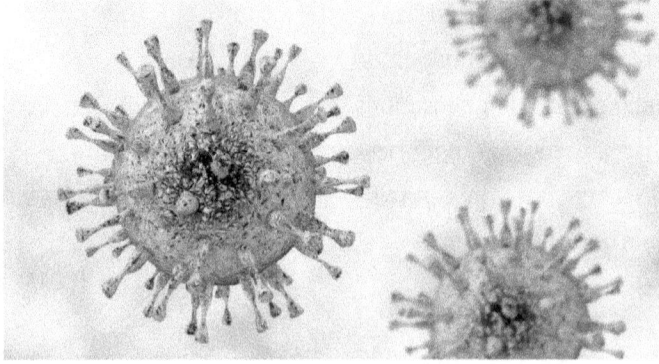

Figure: 19. The genital herpes virus causes sore spots and some swelling

Many of the African Australians as well as some Anglo-Australians do not know about genital herpes and as a result may ask "What is genital herpes?" The simplest way we can explain genital herpes is by saying it is a sexually transmitted disease. It causes herpes sores, which are painful blisters (fluid-filled bumps) that can break open and ooze.

In addition, many people don't know what is vaginal or penis thrush. Thrush is an infection with a fungus; it is also known as a yeast infection. The fungus, called candida, occurs naturally in the body, particularly in warm, moist areas such as the mouth and genitals.

Vaginal thrush is a common yeast infection that affects most women at some point. It may be unpleasant and uncomfortable, but can usually be treated with medication. However, for some women, vaginal thrush can be difficult to treat and keeps coming back.

The symptoms of vaginal thrush include the following: -

▶ Itching and soreness around the entrance of the vagina
▶ Vaginal discharge, this is usually odourless and may be thick and white or thin and watery
▶ Pain during sex, which may make a woman worry about having sex
▶ A stinging sensation when urinating
▶ Sometimes the skin around the vagina can be red, swollen or cracked

What should a woman do to reduce vaginal thrush?

Once if a woman knows she gets thrush, the following suggestions may help her to reduce it occurring. She needs to frequently: -

- ▶ Clean the vulva with water and moisturiser soap more than twice a day.
- ▶ Apply a moisturiser to the skin around the vagina several times a day to protect it.
- ▶ Avoid potential irritants in perfumed soaps, shower gels, vaginal deodorants, wipes and douches.
- ▶ Avoid wearing tight-fitting underwear or tights; some women find that special silk underwear designed for people with eczema and thrush is helpful.
- ▶ Ensure your blood pressure is kept under control, if you have diabetes.

What are some of the things that could cause swelling in the vagina?

From the medical point of view, there are many things that could cause swelling in the vagina, and because of the scope of this research and due to lack of space in this book, we are not going to discuss all of them. However, below are some of the things that could cause swelling in the vagina: -

Bacterial Vaginosis can cause swelling in the vagina. The infection occurs when the bacterial inside the vagina becomes disrupted. Having sex with a male partner can disrupt the balance of bacteria in the vagina, which may put a woman at risk of infection. The bacterial communities of healthy vaginas tend to be dominated by one type of bacteria. Women with higher levels of other bacteria are more likely to get urinary tract infections, or even give birth prematurely. Study shows that the condition does not always come with itching or pain but can create a strong fishy smell. It can also cause a grey/white discharge and discomfort during sex.

Rough sex can cause swelling in the female genital area; a vagina can swell when it experiences a trauma. A woman can also experience swelling if she is not properly aroused during sex. The swelling does not need treatment.

Lervicitis herpes can also cause swelling in the vagina. Herpes is highly contagious and always caused by the herpes simplex virus (HSV), which triggers painful blisters.

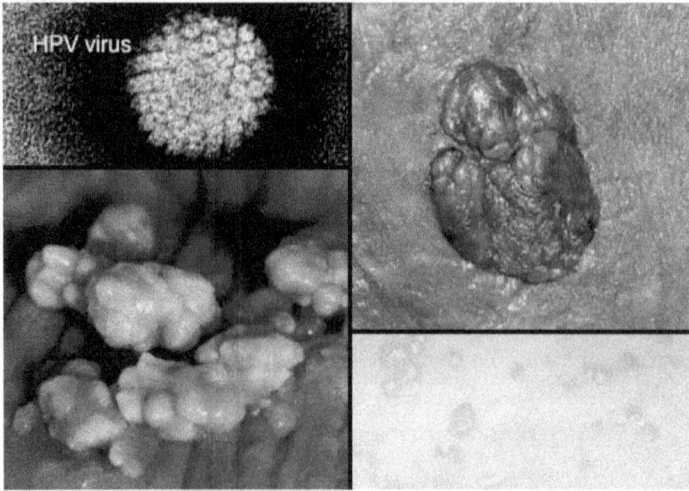

Figure: 20. Herpes Simplex Virus

It is reported that an inflamed cervix or cervicitis is often the result of STI. What is cervicitis? Cervicitis is inflammation of the cervix, which can be due to irritation, infection or injury of cells that line the cervix.

Herpes is spread by skin-to-skin contact, during vaginal, oral or anal sex or even just a kiss. There are two types of herpes, that is HSV1 and HSV2, which enter the body via the skin around the mouth, penis, vagina and rectum. The two types of herpes HSV1 and HSV2 cause cold sores on the mouth, genital herpes and small abscesses on the fingers and hands. The STI caused by herpes virus can cause some swelling and discomfort in women's and man's private parts, it also causes pain while urinating. (Andrea Downey, 2018).

The inflamed cervix causes swelling in the vagina and it also produces pains in the pelvic area; and sometimes cervicitis may cause bleeding and spotting between periods.

Female Reproductive System

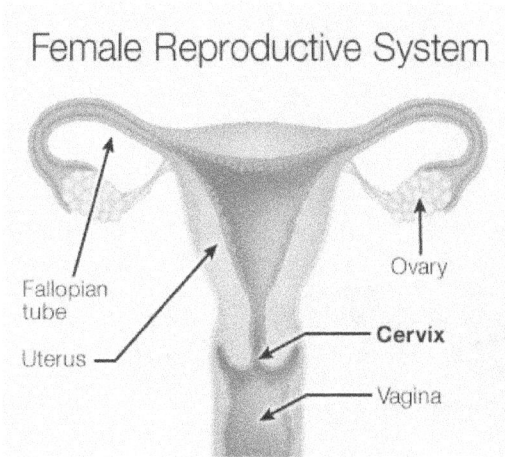

Figure 21. Inflamed Cervix

Determining the cause of cervicitis is important, if an infection is the problem, it can spread beyond the cervix to the uterus and fallopian tubes and into the pelvic area causing swelling and severe pain. Common things that caused cervicitis include gonorrhoea, chlamydia, genital herpes, trichomoniasis, mycoplasma and urea plasma.

One can also bruise the cervix during sex, causing pain and swelling. Experts have found that cycling can be harmful, although it seems like a healthy option, but pedalling could cause swelling around the vagina. According to varies studies conducted in the USA about women who are cycling, they discovered that when a woman sits on a road bike, her vulva, which is not absolutely designed for weight bearing, would be required to take as much as 40 percent of her body weight. This pressure can cause the vulva and labia to appear bigger and become swollen.

Thrush in Men

Thrush is an infection with a fungus and is sometimes known as "yeast infection". It is caused by candida and it occurs naturally in the body particularly in warm, moist areas such as the mouth and genitals. Some heterosexual men get a mild form of balanitis, which is the inflammation of the head of the penis after having sex. This is probably caused by an allergy to the candida fungus in a woman's vagina.

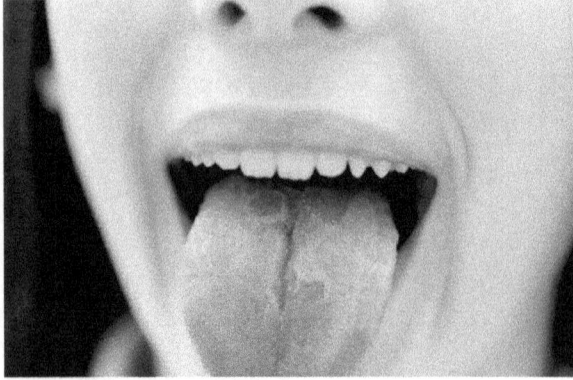

Figure: 22. Yeast infection on the tongue

Symptoms of Thrush in Men

The most common symptoms of thrush in men include: -

- ▶ A very itchy, red and sore head of the penis (glands)
- ▶ Discharge from penis
- ▶ Pain when passing urine
- ▶ Difficulty pulling back foreskin from the penis
- ▶ A cheese-like substance that smells yeasty and sometimes collects under the foreskin of a penis.

However, in some men, thrush also causes the foreskin to swell and crack, which may be caused by an allergy to the yeast. The following are groin irritations experienced by men which are painful and annoying, and are mainly cause by: -

- ▶ Getting sand in a man's shorts or underwear
- ▶ A build-up of sweat after exercise
- ▶ Excess rubbing of the area through sex
- ▶ Lubricants and spermicides
- ▶ Latex products, for example a condom

- Soaps, shower gels, shampoos or hygiene sprays
- Disinfections, antiseptic and ointments
- Washing powders
- New underwear, especially if it is not made from cotton.

Thrush in Women

Thrush is a very common vaginal infection, which is usually caused by an over-growth of yeast which lives normally in the bowel and may be present in other parts of the body, such as mouth, skin and vagina. The most common cause of thrush in both men and women is candida albicans, but other types of yeast may also be involved. Candida is usually present in small numbers and does not show any symptoms. It is only when an overgrowth of candida occurs that symptoms may develop. However, some women are more sensitive than others to the presence of candida, and for this reason, they can develop symptoms even though only small amounts of yeast are present.

Thrush is not considered to be a sexually transmitted infection. The yeast which causes thrush may be present all the time. It is changes in the woman's body which allow the condition to develop.

Signs and symptoms of thrush in women

The symptoms of thrush in women include the following: -

- Vaginal itch, discomfort or irritation
- Vaginal discharge
- Redness and swelling on the vagina or vulva
- Stinging or burning when passing urine

Note well that other conditions, such as vaginal herpes or urinary tract infection may have similar symptoms as we have discussed previously. It is reported that once a woman acquires thrush, she needs to get treatment, but the male partner would not necessarily needs treatment unless the woman has recurrent infections.

Why the Vagina might get hurt during sex?

Some African people are too rough in sex because they think that a vagina can't be hurt. And when you ask them why, they cannot explain the reason, which means they act on assumptions. However, scholars have discovered that there are reasons why we can say certainly that a vagina may be hurt during sex. According to Caroline Kee (2018), sex can hurt people both physiologically and psychologically. Penetrative sex can sometimes be uncomfortable and sometimes it really hurts. The medical term for penetrative sex is "dyspareunia", which refers to re-occuring or persistent pain before, during, or after sex. The pain might only occur upon entry, as the penis enters the vagina and with deep thrusting the level of pain could range from mild to severe. And it can be very frustrating when something that's supposed to be pleasurable causes pain and discomfort instead.

Thus, in this book, we attempt to answer the question, "What can cause painful sex?" And for the purpose of our targeted audience (i.e. African Australians and others who may be interested), we are going to focus on what causes pain in penetrative vaginal sex, which means sex involving a penis or finger going into the vagina. For us to understand the subject better, we shall view the topic under the following six sub-headings: -

> ► An active vaginal infection: When a woman has an active infection, such as genital herpes (see Figure 21 above), UTIs, yeast infections, chlamydia and gonorrhoea, all these can cause pain in penetrative vaginal sex; subsequently, it can make sex painful and uncomfortable. These infections can cause inflammation or irritation of the vulva and vaginal canal, which makes entry and penetration really hurt. Some infections can also affect the cervix and uterus, which may cause deeper with deeper thrusting.

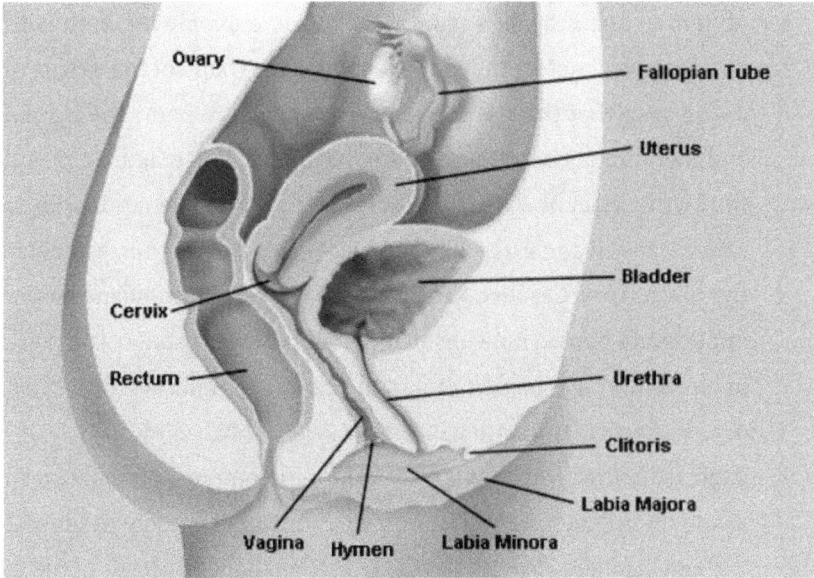

Figure: 23. Areas where vaginal infections can happen

▸ Caroline Kee (2018) observes that the skin of the vulva and vaginal opening is not uncommon where injuries occur. There are many factors that could cause these injuries — these may include an accident, surgery, pelvic trauma, female circumcision, or an incision made to widen the birth canal (episiotomy). They can cause tears and eventually make sex very painful upon entry, especially if there is a wound that is not fully healed.

▸ The vagina is an elastic, muscular canal with a soft, flexible lining that provides lubrication and sensation. The vagina connects the uterus to the outside world. The vulva and labia form the entrance and the cervix of the uterus protrudes into the vagina, forming the interior end. The vagina receives the penis during sexual intercourse and serves as a conduit for the menstrual flow from the uterus. During childbirth, the baby passes through the vagina what is usually called birth canal. The hymen is a thin membrane of tissue that surrounds and narrows the vaginal opening. It may be torn or ruptured by sexual activity or by exercise.

► Abnormal anatomy: It is reported that some people are born with an anatomical defect that either changes the shape of the vagina or makes it so that there is little or no opening. We know the hymen and membrane that covers the vaginal opening (see figure 24), and the myths about how it breaks during intercourse. Therefore, when a woman has an abnormal anatomy this can cause her pain in penetrative vaginal sex. Caroline Kee (2018) argues, "When someone has an imperforate hymen it means that the membrane is abnormally thick or bleeds during their period, and the blood can collect in the vagina". And this can cause pain in penetrative vaginal sex.

► Vaginal dryness: When sex is painful during penetration, it could mean a woman isn't sufficiently lubricated. Moisture is the key to sex and without it, penetrative sex can cause friction that often leads to micro-tears and irritation. According to Caroline Kee (2018), vaginal dryness could be caused by a change or suppression of hormones, which can happen during pregnancy, menopause or when a woman is on birth control. Stress can also change the body's chemistry and result in a loss of moisture. Medications, such as antidepressants and antihistamines like Benadryl, can cause vaginal dryness. Subsequently, when a woman has a dry vagina during sexual intercourse this can cause pain in penetrative vaginal sex.

► Not enough lubricant: Study shows that vaginal dryness is not only caused by hormones and medications, as we have discussed above, but sometimes the lubricant in a woman's vagina isn't enough to last throughout sex, which can lead to discomfort, friction, and pain during penetration or deep thrusting. So, a woman needs enough vaginal lubricant to avoid pain — in this case lubrication should be her really best friend. She can use "lube" during foreplay and penetration, it will keep the vagina moist, and if the lube is not good enough, she can try another type and see which one works better. The following vaginal friendly lubes could be worth trying e.g. Vagisil Prohydrate,

Internal Moistening Gel, Leo Personal Lubricant, Uber Lube, Bezwecken OstaDermV and BeeFriendly.

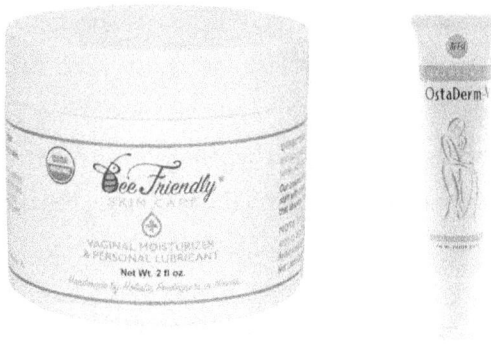

Figure: 24. BeeFriendly and OstaDermV Lubricants

▶ From all the types of lubricants I have mentioned above, it appears "Bezwecken OstaDermV and BeeFriendly are the best treatment of vagina dryness. If a woman wants to use Bezwecken OstaDermV, she should apply one quarter of a teaspoon on the vulva to replace natural lubrication. It is said that many women have praised Bezwecken OstaDermV for not only allowing them to have sex, but to enjoy it again. Study revealed that when women get older their vaginas dry out from the inside and having sex can be difficult. Thus Bezwecken OstaDermV helps to balance woman's hormones. Similarly, BeeFriendly is one of the best lubricants a woman can use. It is made with anti-inflammatory and antimicrobial organic ingredients that work to reduce irritation, itchiness, redness and burning. It does not treat a yeast infection, but it does treat dryness and irritation in the vagina.

▶ These vagina-friendly lubes are equivalent to male erection; the woman needs stimulation and foreplay, or else sex is probably going to be uncomfortable or painful. The vagina is self-lubricating, but it takes a little work and dedication to get the liquids flowing. It takes a woman's body at least twenty minutes to become fully aroused, which includes engorgement of erectile tissue in the labia, clitoris and vaginal canal. (Caroline Kee, 2018). Betty Dodson (2011) argues that for most women to become fully aroused would ideally require clitoral stimulation for at least 30 minutes or even more. When this happens, the uterus lifts (called ballooning) and creates more space, which adds another inch or two in depth that would allow deeper penetration.

► However, it has been reported by some African men that some African women don't want stimulation (by engorging the clitoris) as well as foreplay. They associate engorging of the clitoris and foreplay with prostitution. More importantly, it appears these are the women who experience pain during sex, and they don't like to complain. However, life is changing for some African Australians, it is reported that some women prefer stimulation and foreplay, and they always ask their partners to give them more time before sexual intercourse. It has also been reported that some African Australians do rush into penetrative sex which often makes sex uncomfortable for some women. Therefore, this book wants to inform African Australians that slowing things down and being more mindful about foreplay and sexual arousal can really help in your relationships.

► Certain Positions: Many African Australian women I have spoken to in my research, reported that they feel perfectly fine and good in some positions they use in sex, but other positions cause them lots of pain during penetration and deep thrusting. When I heard that, I then thought to myself, "A couple should always find a good position which is comfortable for both, because anatomy is unchangeable. My people should put shame aside and approach their doctors to explain the situation, and I am sure the doctor can help the couple find a suitable position that works for their bodies." Therefore, a bad position can cause pain in penetrative vaginal sex.

► Can all vaginas handle a big penis: Caroline Kee (2018) observes that a large penis or dildo (within a reasonable size range) can also cause discomfort and pain, but it is highly unlikely that a penis is too big for any vagina or that it will injure the cervix. If a woman's vagina can accommodate a baby's head that is 10 centimetres in diameter, how come that a vagina cannot accommodate a big penis? There is no penis in the world that measures 10 centimetres in diameter — like the head of a baby. Betty Dodson (2011) also observes that there are some women who naturally have deep vaginas; and for the most part, 10 to 12 inch penises are only prized in porn. Most smart men with very large penises know to be gentle and not drive it in "up to the hilt". Overall we can say that the vagina of a woman has a collapsed space that can accommodate any sized penis. However, even though the vagina of a woman can accommodate a big penis, it can cause pain in penetrative vaginal sex.

▶ Psychological Factors: Fear and anxiety around penetration can create a mental barrier which can lead a woman to unconsciously tense-up her pelvic floor muscles during sex and this can cause a physical barrier of penetration. Some scholars said that some women have had a negative sexual experience, so when they are at the point of having sex, they anticipate pain and discomfort. Such women might have experienced trauma such as sexual abuse, violation of boundaries, or sexual assault. As a result, the mind can go into panic. It is also reported that poor self-esteem and body image issues can also decrease arousal or cause someone to become tense or nervous during sex. According to Wright LaNika L. (2019), sexual victimization is a major issue across the globe, especially in America. The results of sexual victimization can persist throughout life and can be debilitating. Sexual victimization affects mental, sexual, and physical health.

▶ Can a penis get stuck in a vagina? According to some scholars, very few reports have documented the existence of a penis having been stuck in a vagina. This is due to the outcome of a condition that is called medically as "vaginismus", in which the vagina involuntarily closes due to muscles spasms in the pelvic floor. How can it occur? Penis captivus is a rare occurrence during sexual intercourse when the muscles in the vagina clamp down on the penis much more firmly than usual, making it impossible for the penis to be withdrawn from the vagina. Jon Johnson (2019) noted that the vaginal walls are made up of muscular tissue, which expands and contracts at different times during sex, such as during an orgasm. These contractions can be very strong, and sometimes may even be stronger than usual. In some rare cases, the vagina may contract with enough force to latch onto the penis, and could make it difficult for the couple to separate. Although penis captivus is a rare occurrence, it can cause pain in penetrative vaginal sex.

▶ However, when these vaginal constrictions come to an end, the vaginal walls will relax; the blood will eventually flow away from the penis, the penis will become smaller and softer, and when this happens the penis will come out of the vagina and the couple would separate. The time it takes for the penis to become smaller and softer varies from person to person.

▶ Therefore, when either partner feels penis captivus is almost starting, they should stay calm because adding stress can lead to more muscular tension and can make the phenomenon last longer. Taking deep breaths may help both partners to remain calm and allow the muscles in both bodies to relax and help resolve the issue as soon as possible without complication. Thus, when you get stuck, do not try to open the vagina or pry the penis out manually.

▶ We have just examined above that a vagina can involuntarily close due to muscles spasms in the pelvic floor. In addition, I want to reassure readers that spasms can make activities such as inserting tampons difficult or impossible. The spasms can also interrupt penetrative sex or make it uncomfortable for either or both parties. But many people still question, "Can it really happen?"

▶ According to Jon Johnson (2019), there are few credible reports of a penis getting stuck in a vagina. Some people, including medical doctors, question if it really exists. There are no well-documented cases. However, there was a review in the BMJ in 1979 that notes that the penis getting stuck in the vagina is factual; the author of the article concludes that although penis captivus may seem to be a myth, medical doctors have reported it. The lack of medical documentation may stem from the temporary nature of the phenomenon. If penis captivus was routinely severe enough to require medical attention, it would likely have inspired more reporting.

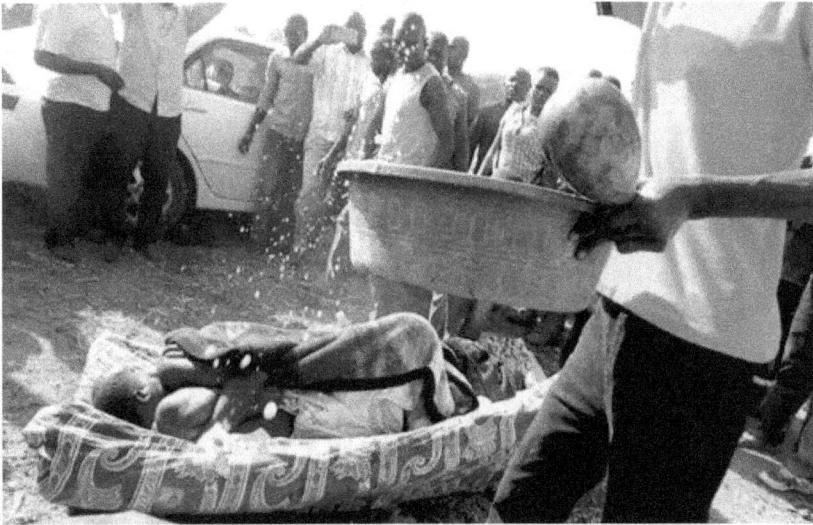

Figure: 25. Penis Captivus is so rare.

► Even though many people do not believe that a penis can get stuck in a vagina, it is reported that if penis captivus occurs, the effect is likely to be very temporary. Should this happen to you one night, the best advice for you and your partner is to relax and give it some time, the muscles should relax, and eventually you will separate. There is no need to raise alarm at this point. One of the medical doctors responded in 1980 to the 1979 review and he wrote to the BMJ to confirm the existence of penis captivus. He said in his letter that in 1979 a young couple were taken to the hospital by ambulance because they were stuck.

▶ William Kremer (2014) reported in BBC News Magazine that penis captivus sounds like a scene from a trashy sex comedy, but the reality is that the stories of a penis getting stuck in a vagina during sex have been with us for centuries. And to substantiate his argument, he quoted one woman writer as saying, "I must tell you the truth, it is no myth. It happened to my late husband and myself one night. He literally could not withdraw his penis from my vagina — we were stuck. I attributed it to the intensity of my vaginal muscle response during orgasm". Recently there were media reports of penis captivus in Kenya, Malawi, Zimbabwe and the Philippines, (no report yet in Australia). The Kenya incident was in 2012; the incident in Zimbabwe was in 2013 that a woman was bringing a law case against her long-term boyfriend for putting a substance known locally as "runyoka" on her — a fidelity spell that caused her to get stuck to her other lover. She was demanding compensation from the jealous boyfriend for humiliating her and for trying to control how she should use her private part. Therefore, we cannot rule out that penis captivus cannot happen.

The average size of a penis

When I was still a young man in Africa, we used to go for bath in the river. As we were naked in the water, some of us wondered why we did not have same sized penis; some had a short penis and others had an extraordinary long-sized penis. This made some of us ask, "Is my penis length normal? Do I have the right sized penis? None of us found an answer to this question. However, in this book I want to inform our African men, both young and old, that those who want to know what the average penis length could be, you should understand that there is a slight deviation between what we men think is normal and what might be the average. Modern studies show that penis size, on an average, is not as big as we men think.

Scientists and psychologists found that penis size is a common source of anxiety for men. There are many factors that can contribute to the anxiety that makes a man think that his penis is smaller than the average man's, and this can make him worry if his penis is really satisfying his partner. However, the truth is that although penis size is dependent on various anatomical factors, in addition to body dysmorphic disorder in men of all ages, all these create a distorted perception of what is *normal*.

A study was conducted in 2015 among 15,521 men; all of them were flaccid and fully erect. It turns out that from these fully erect penises, the average penis size falls somewhere between 4 — 6 inches, with many 5.16 inches long, with penis circumference measuring around 4.5 inches (see Figure: 27 below). The study also found that the average penis length varied from country to country with Poland, Australia and Germany polling the highest, with most men averaging to around 6.14 inches. It was also found that participants involved in the study overestimated the average penis size by about half an inch to one inch (timesofindia.com 2019). It was unfortunate that African men were not included in this study, should they have been included, I am 99.9% sure that they would have been among the men averaging 6.14 inches. Although people from some races around the world were not included in the survey, the reality is that the average penis size (when erect) is somewhere between 5 and 6 inches.

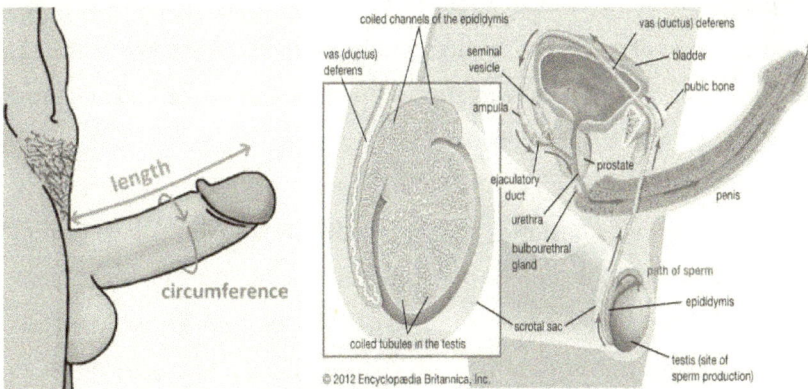

Figure 26. Length and Figure: 27. Channels for ejaculation
& circumference of an erect penis
Sources: Encyclopædia Britannica, Inc.

Therefore, it is recommended that one should not worry whether his penis is good enough or promising enough for his sexual partner; there is no point in comparing oneself with another, as long as your penis is functioning well, there is no need to bother with such trivialities.

No matter what size of penis a man has, the penis has the capability to pleasure and satisfy his partner and his performance does not depend on his penis (short or long) but it rather depends on techniques, movements, and positions a man and a woman have at the time of intercourse.

Penile Erection

Before sex, the penis is normally erect, which is given the noun "erection" and is also called *Penile Erection*. Erection in human terms is known as an enlargement, hardening, and elevation of the male penis. (See Figure 28: structures involved in the production and transport of semen). Internally, the penis has three long masses of cylindrical tissue, known as erectile tissue, that are bound together by fibrous tissue. The two identical areas running along the sides of the penis are termed corpora cavernosa; the third mass, known as the corpus spongiosum that lies below the corpora cavernosa, and is surrounded by the urethra, extends forward to form the tip (or glands) of the penis (See Figure 29 below). All three masses are spongelike; they contain large spaces between loose networks of tissue. The corpus spongiosum does not become as erect as the corpora cavernosa. The veins are more peripherally located, so that there is a continual outflow of blood in this region.

When the penis is in a flaccid or resting state, the spaces collapse, and the tissue is condensed. And during erection, blood flows into the spaces, causing distention and elevation of the penis, (See figure 27). The amount of blood entering the penis can be increased by physical or psychological stimulation. As blood enters, there is a temporary reduction in the rate and volume of blood leaving the penis. The arteries carrying blood to the penis dilate; this in turn, causes tissue expansion. The veins leading from the penis have funnel-shaped valves that reduce the outflow of blood. As the erectile tissue begins to enlarge, the additional pressure causes the veins to be squeezed against the surrounding fibrous tissue, and this further diminishes the outflow of blood. Essentially, blood becomes temporarily trapped in the organ.

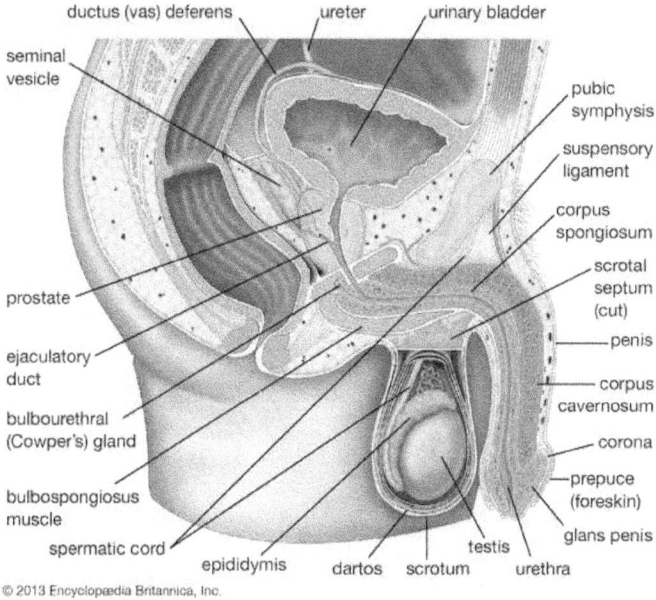

Figure: 28. Male reproductive system

Chapter Six
Dating And Remarriage

Can sugar relationships lead to marriage?

When I thought of writing about remarriage among African men and women following sugar relationships, I began to ponder on whether this could happen or not. So, I sent questions to over 80 Africans (both men and women). The question was simple and it says, *"Can a sugar relationship lead to marriage?"* I received mixed responses from the respondents: Some of them stated that a sugar relationship would never lead to marriage, because it is purely based on money and sex — it is just for enjoyment and nothing else. Some said that a sugar relationship could lead to marriage if it is built on real love and not on personal interest, and a member of the party was not playing games. Others said that a sugar relationship would hardly ever lead to marriage. They justified their argument by saying that a sugar relationship follows the natural law of demand and supply. It will only last as long as supply meets demand and until the demanding person is satisfied. And if the money and other materials are not forthcoming, one of the partners (usually a woman) will see no value in the relationship and will bring it to an end. Similarly, if a man sees that his demands are not being met by a sugar baby on a regular basis, he may decide to withdraw from the relationship. In short, a sugar relationship always come to an end in the absence of money and/or sex.

In the research, it was found that there is no indication that sugar relationships among African Australians, would end up in marriage even though some people expected that it could. Research also revealed that a sugar baby with multi-relationships is more unlikely to marry.

Remarriage of divorced mothers/fathers and widows/widowers

"Remarriage following the death of a husband/wife has important implications for an individual woman and man in the States and Territories of Australia. Research in the Caprivi Region of Namibia found that while widowers and single fathers commonly remarry, the traditional option open to women through widow inheritance has been outlived. While forcing widows off the land is now prohibited, socio-cultural pressures, the status of the women's children and a lack of basic support from the late husband's relatives can result in a subtler form of property disinheritance. In addition to upheaval caused by relocation, many widows are limited in understanding livelihood activities, constrained in their capacity to engage in profitable income-earning opportunities, and are heavily reliant on the support of others."

Source: Research by University of Eastern Finland & University of Namibia, 2013.

Marriage or remarriage is teamwork, it requires both partners to put in their individual efforts to make things work. Just as a woman wants a "good husband", the husband would also want a "good wife". How, can we identify a good husband and a good wife from the bad one? The answer to this question may be difficult, but we can find this in Chapter 9.

But before we go deep into the discussion of remarriages, we firstly want to know about the term "widow" "widower" and "widowhood". The term widow is a noun and it means "a woman who has lost her husband by death and is not yet remarried". The term widower is also a noun that means "a man whose wife has died, and he is not yet remarried"; while the state of having lost one's spouse to death is known as widowhood.

Experience tells us that when a woman become a widow, she usually loses family income. For a wife, the death of a husband could change her situation in a moment, but for a widower, his problems could accumulate gradually. Study revealed that when a woman loses her husband, she is deprived of support from traditional forces and this can cause economic hardship or deprivation. The death of a husband, a person considered to be the breadwinner in a family, can cause a breakdown in the family division of labour because she will be taking over roles traditionally carried out only by men.

General talks among the Africans in Australia show that the majority of widows are not ready for remarriage after the death of their husbands, but what they want is only financial support through sugar relationships. This argument can be supported by one true case story from two partners who do not want their names to be disclosed. The story was told to me by a man who preferred to be called Mr Johnson and his sugar baby to be called Ms Rose Mary for the purpose of confidentiality and privacy. The man also advised not to mention the location where they live, otherwise it may create suspicion among the Africans.

Finding a husband is hard, however, the following wise saying tell us that if:

- You find a handsome one, the brain is empty
- You find a brilliant one. He may look too serious in all situations
- You find a rich one, he is sometimes may be disgraceful
- You find a hard-working one, he may not have time for you
- You find a serious one, his Exs may keep calling you or him on mobile
- You find a humble one, he may be literally broken
- You find a responsible one, he may not be romantic
- You find an educated one, he may feel he is always right, and you are always wrong
- You find an illiterate one, he may always get angry whenever you correct him
- You find a smart one, he may be telling you lies every time

A true Scenario of Mr Johnson and Ms Rose Mary

The story of the two couples demonstrates how sugar babies and sugar daddies think differently when it comes to remarriage and more importantly, when it comes to the matter of being honest or dishonest about remarriage. From the narrative we are made to understand that a man wants sex and remarriage eventually, but a widow only wants financial support in addition to sexual enjoyment. Mr Johnson is a divorced husband and has three children with his former wife. The children are with their mother. Ms Rose Mary is a widow who lost her husband and does not want to be inherited by the brother or male cousin of the dead husband.

Mr Johnson said that one Sunday evening they were together in a motel. He said he has been in a sugar relationship with Rose Mary for ten years and during this time he has discovered that the woman does not like to open her heart to him. Mr Johnson said from day one, he told his woman that he was not looking for a child or children in their relationship, but he is looking for love and remarriage. After four years of relationship, one day he asked her if they could get married. The woman said, "Please, give me time. I want time to think about it and I will get back to you with an answer."

Mr Johnson said, "Although we meet regularly, I waited for the response from the woman for three months and to my surprise, there was no answer. I started to feel that she is dishonest, and is a more money and material-minded person."

Mr Johnson told me that he could not make up his final decision for remarriage until he received approval from Rose Mary, which would mean they have the same values and aspirations.

Mr Johnson said as they were sitting in their motel room, he decided to ask Rose Mary three basic questions. He thought that by answering these questions honestly, he may get to know and understand her better since he was already losing his patience. The questions were as follows: —

Mr Johnson: "Please, Rose Mary, can you tell me three things you like most during our ten years of relationship?

Ms Rose Mary, "The three things I like most during our ten years of relationship are:

▶ I like the way we play sex; I have enjoyed nearly 75% of sexual intercourse with you.

▶ I like seeing you upset whenever I cancel or change our appointments.

▶ I like the way you support me financially and materially. You are always helpful whenever I am in financial hardship and you have been behind me through out these periods.

Mr Johnson: "Please, list three things your dislike about our relationship".

Ms Rose Mary, "Why are you asking me these questions? I don't want to answer this second question because when I answer it would make me recall our past misunderstandings".

Mr Johnson: "I understand where you are coming from, but the reality is that the answers to all these questions would help us improve our relationship. We all learn through mistakes". So, she was convinced and answered the questions as follows:

Ms Rose Mary: "The three things I disliked during our ten years of relationship include:

▶ The ways you often don't like my suggestions which caused many disagreements.

▶ The way you treated me when I went overseas (to Africa) in 2017; you did not send me some financial assistance when I was in much need of funds.

▶ The way you withheld your full financial and material support by nearly half in the last three years. In the beginning of our relationship, you used to support me fully, which made me happy. You have stopped giving me Christmas gifts, although you still give some funds for Christmas. You should not expect support from me, but I instead expect support from you."

Mr Johnson: "Please can you list three things we should do to improve our relationship?"

Ms Rose Marry: "How can you fix what has happened in past? This question makes me recall many things about our relationship. I don't want to talk about the past."

Mr Johnson: "As I told you before, we all learn from our past mistakes, but we cannot go back and fix what has been done wrongly in the past. More importantly, talking about the past can help us identify our past weaknesses, and it can act as a tool to construct a better road for our future life.

Ms Rose Mary: "You know what happened with our relationship in the past. Therefore, what I want is that *you must change.*"

Mr Johnson: "As human beings, I know both of us have made mistakes in the past; and in this case, making a change is not one-way traffic. This implies that you and I might have done something wrong in the past, which might have caused some inconvenience to each one of us. Therefore, both of us may need to change as the years are passing."

Ms Rose Mary: "To the best of my knowledge, you were making many mistakes in the past, especially during the last five years of our relationship. On my side, I know I have done nothing wrong."

Mr Johnson: "I am a bit disappointed with your cancelation of our appointments during the past ten years. Why you do not stick to the appointments?"

Ms Rose Mary: "My dear, I am too busy. I have many visitors besides my domestic work."

Mr Johnson: "Time can be good, and it can also be bad, depending on the way you manage it. Time is powerful; it can determine your past as well as your future. Don't allow your emotions to control you. God has given us time for a purpose, that is, for us to use it to achieve our goals. Make time for your friends and manage it. Use time to benefit you and your partner. Look to the future and don't confine yourself to the present. You have power to recreate yourself and redesign your day. Do something, get on track, and keep your love moving in the right direction."

Ms Rose Mary: "What you are saying, are all nonsense."

Mr Johnson: "Darling, no one is an angel under the sun. However, what is the way forward? Where are we leading to with our relationship?"

Ms Rose Mary: "I don't want to answer this question because you kept on bringing it up again and again. I thought I have been very clear to you about our relationship. If you don't remember, what I want in our relationship is that you and I must be safe from the tongues of the community. I also want respect for our children. I have collected enough information about you from your past mistakes. I now know your feelings; I also now know why you have withdrawn full financial and material support from me."

Mr Johnson: "You have never been clear to me. I asked you five years ago whether you would like to remarry me. You told me to give you time to think it over and you would get back to me. Up-to-date you did not do this. What does this mean for our relationship? I told you from day one that if our relationship grows well and healthy and makes us realise that we have the same values, I would then like to remarry you."

Ms Rose Mary: "I now understand why you do not want to fully support me. I have asked many things from you and you have turned down my requests. I know you did not want to supply me with these things because I am not ready for remarriage, and in addition, I have had no child with you during the last five years."

Mr Johnson: "Why don't you want to remarry me?"

Ms Rose Mary: "I am not ready for remarriage, but I am happy the way we have been. I know you have been divorced, but I am a woman and I know what women think and can do even after divorce. Women are the same. Therefore, if I accepted to remarry you, your ex-wife will come to fight me in our new house, and she will find ways to destroy our relationship. This is the thing I don't want to happen in my remaining lifetime. It is better for us to remain the way we are; you continue to support me, and we continue to meet in our agreed place for sex — and that is all."

Mr Johnson: "Darling, we do not have the same values and aspirations. When I met you, I thought at the end I would remarry you."

Ms Rose Mary, "I love you because I believe it's a blessing from God and you will support me. For this reason, I have given you my body. Because I strongly believe that you will rescue me from my past sufferings".

Mr Johnson, "I also believe our love has come from God. So, let's enjoy peace of minds and hearts. You are the Queen of my heart. I love you so much".

Ms Rose Mary, "I love you too; nevertheless, after eight years of our sexual relationship, I have now started to develop low moral about our relationship. As such, I have decided that today should be our last day for our sexual meeting. I want you to leave me alone for three months, I have something disturbing me in my heart. I want to remove that thing from my heart, and this may enable me to reconsider your proposal for remarriage".

Mr Johnson, "Are you asking for a break because you want to make up your mind of "who" to choose from among men with whom you are in relationship?"

Ms Rose Mary, "No. I don't have other men to choose from, but I just want a break. I am a woman who can engage man, but a man cannot engage me".

Mr Johnson, "OK! I can't stand on your way. I respect your opinion, and I wish you all the best during your three-month break. However, I want to inform you that during this three-month break, I am not going to give you the regular financial support".

Ms Rose Mary, after three months Rose Mary and Mr Johnson met in their usual place (Motel). Rose Marry said to Johnson, "Thank you for our eight years of sugar relationship. Many things have happened during our love. I have taken a three-month leave by myself because first I want to examine myself and secondly, I want to see how you would react about my decision. So, I want you to answer these three questions: (1) How did you feel when I took that leave from sexual relationship? (2) What do you think about me during the last three months of leave? (3) Can you continue to be my friend but with less demands for sexual intercourse?

Mr Johnson, "I respect your opinions. True and sincere love is something that is very precious, and no one can buy it with money. If a person buys a true and genuine love with money, and tomorrow when there is no money this so-called love will come to an end -this is a material love. Road to remarriage is rough and narrow.

Ms Rose Mary, "I have something big in my heart, and I have no courage to say it out".

Mr Johnson, "If you sincerely love and trust me, why don't you open your heart to me? Those questions may sound a bit silly, but they are the core of our love. We should understand that love can be defined as happiness, comfort, relaxation, perfect harmony. True lovers are opened to one another as well as caring for each other.

Ms Rose Mary, "We all have children, and we are talking about remarriage. We need to discuss about the children and how they would react to our remarriage. Secondly, I know, I have often turned down our appointments. In the last ten years of our sugar relationship, we have had 240 appointments for sexual relationship, out of these, I have accepted 120 appointments (in ten years). The reasons for turning down the appointments were many and these includes being too busy, funerals, community meetings, lunch with friends in hotels, travelling outside my suburb, having visitors and going out to visit my relatives and friends. I know you were not happy about my rejection of the appointments -I am sorry dear.

Mr Johnson, "It is true that both of us have children, but what I want to know is that, are you ready to remarry me?"

Ms Rose Mary, "Why do you keep on asking same question over and over? We have already reached an agreement on the matter".

Mr Johnson, "In which way did we reach the agreement? You told me in the past that you were going to think about it — on whether you accept remarriage or not".

Ms Rose Mary, "At his time, I cannot say to you Yes or No. When times comes, I will let you know. It is not difficult to make my decision. All of us know a "decision' can be made *for* or *against*".

Mr Johnson After two months, Mr Johnson asked Rose Mary again, "My sweetheart, I have been asking you this question over and over, yet without answer: What is going on in your mind right now? Are your ready to remarry me?"

Ms Rose Mary "Stop pushing me in sex and to make decision; I am not ready for -remarriage. Why do you ask, "What is in my mind?" You already know what is going on in my mind. Please, take me out of your mind at present. Better you give me my freedom. I will call you and tell you when I am ready for remarriage".

Mr Johnson "I am confused, let us suspend the topic for our next meeting (in three days). However, I want to tell you that last week, I have been calling you and you did not pick up my calls. I have also been sending you SMS and you never responded to any of them. I love you and have put my trust in you. Why do you want to turn me down?"

Ms Rose Mary "I cannot response to your statement at this time, but we shall discuss more in our next meeting (in three days)".

Mr Johnson After one day Mr Johnson wanted to visit Rose Marry in her house. He called and asked, "Are you at home"?

Ms Rose Mary "Yes, I am in the house but don't come. I have a visitor in the house. This visitor has never been in my house before".

Mr Johnson "I know you don't want me to come to your house, but can I just come to greet the visitor"?

Ms Rose Mary "No. Please, don't come -if you do not want me to get angry with you".

Mr Johnson "Why should you get angry with me"?

Ms Rose Mary "I have already told you not to come". After the phone conversation there was no phone calls for a week.

Mr Johnson Could not tolerate the situation, he went to consult a lady family friend. When Johnson arrived in the house of family friend, he said to her, "I have a sugar baby whom I want to remarry. We have been in relationship for ten years and approximately three months. My sugar baby has two grown up children one is a girl and the other is a boy. I often visit her in her house and the children know me very well. Last week I wanted to visit my sugar baby in the house, but she advised me that the best time for visit is Monday. We then agreed to meet on Monday at around 5.00 p.m. On Monday, before 5.00 p.m. my sugar baby called and said she would not be at home, and she didn't know at what time she would be at home. I told her, *"I will wait for you in the car outside your house until you come home"*. She responded, *"Don't go and wait for me at home, I have a visitor coming at 5.30 p.m. And if you come, I will be angry with you"*. She then hanged up the phone on my ear. My concerns are these: During our ten years and three months of relationship, our love has been up and down. She did not keep our appointments and she demand more financial and material supports. What does this mean and what can I do to fix the problems?"

Johnson's Family-friend answers "The woman might have other men to attend to. That is why she did not want you to visit her when a visitor was in the house because she does not want you to meet with other men face to face. I tell you, if you want to remarry, this woman cannot make good wife. You better look for another woman for marriage. This woman is just looking for financial and material supports from you. But if you insist to remarry her, do not be in a hurry for otherwise this woman will make you regret in future".

Mr Johnson After one week of meeting a family friend, Mr Johnson went to Rose Mary and asked, "What is your problem? Why did you not like me to visit you when you had a visitor?

Ms Rose Mary "I was disturbed; and why do you insist to come to my house when I have visitors". After this short conversation, there was not sexual relationship for two months; in addition, there were not any communication.

Mr Johnson After two months Mr Johnson called Rose Mary and said, "Darling, my heart is with you. Don't blame your behaviours on other people. You are 100% responsible for our deteriorating relationship -no matter how bad you are feeling or what happen to you.

Ms Rose Mary "Hoo! My sweetheart, I love you can you call me tomorrow?"

Mr Johnson -The following morning Mr Johnson called Rose Mary and said, "Our relationship should be based on trust and royalty. Love is not just a word that a person can just say, "I love you", it is more than that. It is how you can prove to your partner that your love is sincere, genuine and true. This is what I can tell you about love my wife".

Ms Rose Mary "Hey! I am not your wife. We are just friends. Our situation cannot allow us to stay together with you under the same roof".

Mr Johnson "Do you want us to separate from our sugar relationship?"

Ms Rose Mary "No, I don't want us to separate from our sugar relationship, but I want us to continue in the same way we have been for the last ten years and three months. I will never leave you, unless you decide to leave me. You know I am not always happy and often feel distress. You should listen to someone like me with distress. Although I want our sugar relationship to continue -you should know that love is not sexual intercourse it is more to do with helping me in my difficulties".

Mr Johnson "At last, after ten years and three months I have understood you. You want our sugar relationship to continue without any hope for remarriage". I want to ask you, "What will happen if I get remarry to another woman, shall we continue with our relationship?"

Ms Rose Mary "Absolutely, I would not mind you having a wife, in as long as we keep our relationship secret."

Me Johnson "Let us continue with the game in accordance with your plan. However, times will tell how long we shall keep on with such a relationship".

Economic Challenges

Some African Australians have either lost their partners or are divorced, and the divorce rates among African Australians have been going up since 2006. As a matter of fact, life can become unbearable for a surviving spouse, single mother or a widower. Therefore, remarriage is one of the most important determinants of physical and economic wellbeing among them in such a situation. When a spouse has died, after a while one may think about the possibility of remarriage. Although during my research, the case of remarriage was a rare topic of conversation.

However, I felt that I should include the topic of remarriage in this book. This may provide an opportunity to know how many African widows, widowers, single mothers and single fathers are getting remarried in Australia.

It is reported that widowers with three to six children at home have a lower rate of remarriage. Unfortunately, there is no data to back-up this argument. It appears that the widows, widowers, single mothers and single fathers are people between 48 to 60 years. What we know from African Australians is that many children of widows suffer when their father dies, because the single income from the mother cannot cover all the basic needs, given that living costs in Australia are getting higher and higher. Subsequently, single mothers and widows find it difficult to make decisions on what the family should do to survive. Michael J. Brien et al. (2001) observes that economic theory suggests that economic incentives play a role in family structure decision-making. In support of this theory, there is growing evidence that the implicit incentives in government programs for single mothers and widows, affect them in their decision as to whether and when to remarry.

With this economic challenge, some African women believe that one of the options to solve the problems of a single mother and widowhood is to become a sugar baby or to remarry when chances are available. The popular stereotype presents remarriage as the best option for the widow rather than for the single mother. This is a good option for widows who have lost their financial support provided previously by a dead husband. Contrarily, the popular stereotype for divorced wives presents becoming sugar babies as the best option. They often think this way because their ex-husbands, who are living in Australia, could kill the new men. Since the practice of sugar relationships among African Australians is done secretly or underground, this could offer an opportunity to have a sugar daddy who would support them for the rest of their life.

Remarriage by widows appears to reconstruct a family that had been broken by death; a new husband gains a family supplier and childcare, while the wife gains kitchen management and production of children. Historians, especially demographers, have assumed that remarriage compensates for the loss of a spouse. Susan Hart (2009) says, "It is not difficult to see why remarriage might have seemed desirable in the eyes of widows; any widow in any community is of concern to society because in a patriarchal society (like African communities) the loss of a spouse can leave widows and orphans vulnerable to poverty.

In Australia today, Social Security is a key source of financial security for widowed spouses and single mothers. Because of this, many individuals who have lost their spouses receive Social Security Benefits based on different considerations by the Australian Government Department of Human Services (Centrelink). Although Social Security cannot explain why single motherhood is more common among the African Australians.

According to the Australian Government Department of Human Services, Social Security Act 1991, it states that a widow can stay on a widow allowance if she keeps meeting the eligibility criteria. How much widow allowance does a widow usually receives? This depends on her income and assets. The higher the amount she receives from her wages, the less she receives in Social Security payments. Being in a de facto relationship can also reduce Social Security payments. More importantly, the widow may not even receive an allowance at all, if her wages are above the Centrelink required standard.

However, the maximum fortnightly payment for a single mother from Centrelink, without children, is $559.00 and a single mother with children receives $604.70 per fortnight apart from Part B Benefits.

It is stipulated in Government policy that for a single mother with children, she will get the first Widow Allowance for the first nine months, and after the nine months, her Widow Allowance increases from $559 to $604.70. It seems there is no increase in a single mother's payment who has children, because she receives Family Tax Benefit B (this is the payment for children), but we need to confirm this with Centrelink.

With all the above narratives in mind, we should be able to see clearly how difficult it is for a widow to decide whether to remarry or remain receiving Social Security, and at the same time become a sugar baby to get additional funds for her wallet.

We have seen that as African Australians assimilate into Australian society, some of the men started joining the Police Force in different States and

Territories. Some of them are also enrolled in the Army. It was hoped that when these men died, their wives would receive Social Security for their dead spouses. But it is not easy and is more complicated to receive these allowances. The Government has some strings attached to survivor benefits. It is true that when a husband who joined Australian Forces dies, the wife receives a Security Allowance known as "Survivors Annuities", but if a woman decides to remarry, she would lose this benefit.

However, it is stipulated in military law that widows and widowers may lose their annuities when they remarry before the age of 57 (60?), but if they remarry after the age of 57 (60?), they will continue to receive Survivor Benefits. And if a woman was married to the dead husband for at least ten years, and after this she was divorced, if after two years following the divorce the ex-husband dies, she could be eligible for spousal benefits based upon her former husband's record, provided she is still not remarried. (Source: figuide. aom/remarriage rules for widows and widowers 10/11/2019).

Study shows that the negative long-term effects of divorce exist on the relationship between fathers and adult children. Although less often noted, there are also negative effects of divorce on the relationship between children and their mother. However, these effects are smaller in magnitude.

As I mentioned before, there is no data to show how many African Australian widows, widowers, single mothers and single fathers there are. Therefore, it appears that the remarriage rate among the Africans is only 3%.

It is generally believed that when a person's spouse has died, after a period of time a survivor thinks about the possibility of remarriage. The survivor should consider seriously what we are going to discuss in the following subtitle, before deciding, as this may help them make the right decision.

When is the right time to consider remarriage?

There is no one answer to the above question, as it depends on several circumstances. Some people may think that the right time for a widow, widower, single mother and single father to consider remarriage is at least a year following the death or separation of a spouse. However, experiences tell us that if the death of a spouse was sudden, the resolution of grief could take a long time. In this situation, a survivor may find it best to wait for several years before considering remarriage.

Conversely, if a spouse had been suffering illness for a long period of time, one may be comfortable in remarrying in less than a year or so, because that person has gone through a partial process of grief before the death of a mate.

Why do grieving men find lovers faster than grieving widows?

Regardless of race, nationality and culture, widowers seem to become ten times more alluring to the opposite sex, practically overnight, following the death of a wife. But widows are not attracted easily to men in the same way men are attracted to women. Therefore, love after death appears certainly much easier to achieve for men than for women. It seems one of the reasons why is that they do not have close friends with whom they could share ideas, but women have so many friends to talk to; women appear to have a strong emotional support network to help them through bereavement. A recent study found that two-thirds of widowers were in new relationships within 25 months, while less than a fifth of widows are in new relationships within 25 months as opposed to widowers. It is said, over the age of 65, the discrepancy is even larger, with ten times as many widowers as widows remarrying.

Dating after the death of a spouse or after divorce

"The death of spouse has been shown to produce a dramatic decline in the economic and physical wellbeing of the surviving spouse. Yet some widowed individuals can take actions that mitigate these adverse effects. Remarriage is one action that often reduces the surviving spouse's chances of accounting declines in many things." (Helsing and Szklo et al, 1981).

Culturally in Africa, a widow is not allowed to marry a man from outside the family. She is to be inherited by one of the dead husband's brothers in a traditional order. (For more information about inheritance, see *A short Social and Cultural Anthropology of the Northern Luo of South Sudan*, Chapter 22, Author: Saturnino Onyala.)

However, in Australian it is somehow difficult to follow the culture of inheritance, as firstly husbands are not permitted to have two wives, and secondly bringing a brother of the dead husband from Africa to Australia, is difficult. As such, widows are left in a dilemma. So the only option is to date a man from Australia if they want to remarry. Interestingly, when a widow wants to date a man, the period allowed to start dating also varies from community to community. Each African community has a specific period a widow is expected to remarry. After losing someone you loved, the idea of remarrying can be almost unthinkable. In some communities it takes between 1-3 years, but there are some widows who choose not to respect these periods, they attempt to quickly remedy their feelings and find a replacement for a beloved one by between 4 — 6 months. Others choose never to remarry, especially when their children are grown up.

As for divorced women, it is more difficult to find men to remarry. A man who wants to marry a divorced woman must think hard, because you are not sure why she was divorced. What is the guarantee that she will not do the same thing to you, as she has done to her ex-husband? There is a common saying among the Acholi (Luo), which says, "If you find a wood-log on the road, please don't pick it up. If you do, you will not carry it for a long distance, you will throw it down, as the former person has thrown it away because it contains insects that bite. Before long, the insects will also start to bite you and you will throw the wood-log on the road again." This means that once a man marries a divorced woman, they will not live long together. The woman will never change her bad behaviour or bad character. Before long, she will start behaving the same way she did with her former husband and eventually the new husband will be forced to leave her. And the other reason why men do not want to marry divorced wives is because of the fear that their ex-husbands may kill them. For these reasons, a divorced woman remains in the pool of sugar babies until she decides either to reunite with her former husband or to remain in the sugar baby industry for the rest of her life.

"Dipping your toes into the virtual pool can be a terrifying prospect for many seasoned singles, let alone someone taking the first tentative steps towards new love in the wake of a partner's death." By Tome Morrissy, 2017.

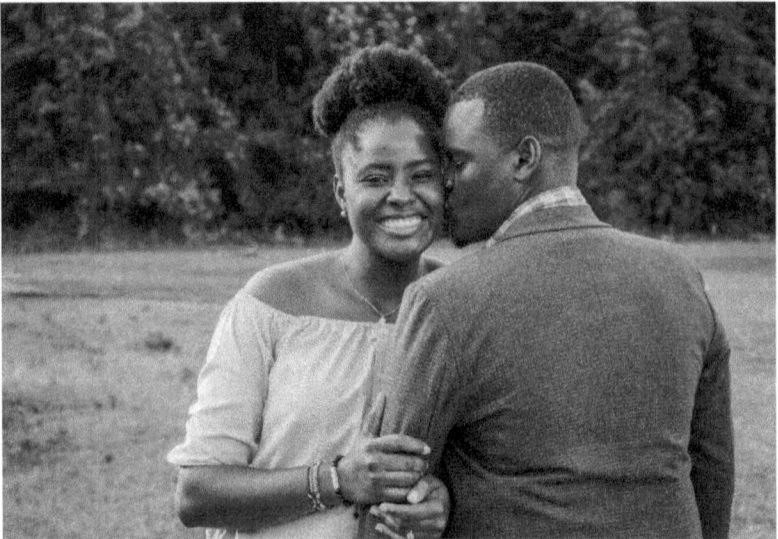

Figure: 29. Dating among African Australians

However, study by some marriage counsellors revealed that widowers and single fathers are more likely to remarry than the divorced wives. In 1996 Annals of Clinical Psychiatry carried out a study among 24 widows and 101 widowers which revealed that 61% of men and 19% of women were remarried by 25 months after a spouse's death.

Let us look back to the Africa continent, as I mentioned before, when a wife loses her husband, the brother of the dead husband will inherit her. Inheritance culture is not acceptable in Australia, so the only option for a widow to maintain herself financially is that she must become a sugar baby. Similarly, for a divorced wife who has lost her husband's income and has to maintain herself and the children financially in Australia, the best option is to become a sugar baby for the rest of her life.

However, it is important to know that finding love and happiness for widows and single mothers again is not about replacing what one had before, or to forget about the last spouse, but rather for economic reasons. As long as a woman lives, she deserves to be happy, and if this means finding a new spouse, then that is welcome.

In Australia there is no set timeframe on when to be ready to find someone, the only issue is who is the right person? You can even decide what the right time to find a new person is. Undocumented statistics show us that today, there are many Africa Australian single mothers, widows, widowers and single fathers, and many of them prefer to marry wives and husbands from overseas. According to men, they prefer to remarry a woman from overseas because they fear that if they remarry a woman from Australia it would be more difficult to handle her than to handle a woman remarried overseas and bought to the country. And for women, they want to remarry a man from overseas because they think it would be easy for them to control the man by threatening him with deportation should he misbehave himself and does not strictly follow what the woman is telling him to do. So, the women think that African men in Australia are sometimes uncontrollable.

However, experiences in Australia tell us that a good number of wives and husbands remarried from overseas, on arrival to Australia, live with the partner while awaiting their Permanent Resident (PR) Visa. In four to six years, when they obtained their PR and citizenship, they immediately divorce the wife or the husband. A man does not think about the difficulties a woman has encountered in bringing him from overseas; and vice versa, a woman she does not think about the difficulties a man has encountered in bringing her from overseas.

For this reason, some of the men prefer to kill their wives and stay in prison for the rest of their lives; in contrast, women find it difficult to kill men, so many of them leave soon after divorce and move to live in another state. Sometimes the African community experiences a woman killed by her husband and not because they are divorced, but rather because a woman may have got pregnant overseas, and on arrival, she declares that she is pregnant by the husband who brought her to the country.

After having said this, I would like to emphasise that some African widows, single mothers and widowers and single fathers enter dating to experience life again and realise that grief and sorrow are holding them back from doing that. Therefore, dating is seen as an adventure and one that evokes so many feelings, as one bravely put himself or herself out there. Once a person is out there, there can be hope, elevation, disappointment, anxiety, frustration and passion. Some of the single mothers are smart, strong and beautiful but also a bit of a mystery. Dating after death or divorce is good, but how can one make this relationship work? And how does a man let his potential partner know that he is not just playing games. Often, when starting to date, many single mothers and widows set the stage for success. Here below are some ways and means for those who want to date and remarry. According to Tome Morrissey Swan (2017) there are thirteen top advices that a person who wants to remarry could follow: -

- ▶ Don't date until you feel ready: In the Africa continent, people mourn for one year and sometimes even more, but in Australia, there is no timeframe for grief. It could take weeks, months or a year, depending on the individual and not on cultures. Don't let people tell you that the right time has come because it is hard to know when you are ready, so don't be afraid.

- ▶ Date for the right reasons: Don't let hardship drive you and don't rush your decision but think carefully why you want to make a relationship again. Otherwise, at the end of the day you will regret it.

- ▶ Be a person of yourself: This may be hard because you have lost part of your identity when your spouse died. So, when you want to make a new relationship, be comfortable and confident in yourself. This will make you more attractive to a potential partner, as well as boosting your own self-esteem.

► Feeling guilty is normal to begin with: You may feel like you are cheating on your ex. You might be embarrassed for your friends and relatives or your ex's friends to know that you are moving toward a new relationship. One of my informants in Australia was telling me that he was in a relationship with a widow who does not want anybody to know. But to make a new relationship is not wrong; if you are ready, don't fear to go on. After a short time, your feelings of guilt will begin to subside.

► Please know that your date is not a therapist: In this case, honesty is crucial; it is not good to hide your ex-spouse or to pretend that you did not love one. It is normal for your potential partner to know you have had a relationship. But don't spend your whole time talking about your ex-friends, because your date is not a therapist as mentioned above. It is better if you focus on the potential person you want to love, and your date is more likely to go well.

► Think of the future: We all have a past, so it doesn't benefit you to dwell on your past, it is usually better to focus on the person you are currently interested in dating. With your partner, think positively and focus more on hopes and dreams of your future, consider what is it that you want from life with this new person, who is here now with you, then move forward.

► Don't rush into your new relationship: Losing a wife or a husband is a huge shock to the family system. You may think of having your previous life with your spouse again, but even though building your new relationship with your new partner is going well, do not try to rush it. Thus, waiting to see if you are not just attempting to replace those feelings of being close to someone again will be better for both sides in a long run. In other words, give your relationship time to develop. Don't rush into moving in to living together or getting engaged. Instead, take it slow and focus on developing trust before you take your relationship to the next level. A good example is that a friend was telling me that he has a new relationship with a woman who is divorced. The relationship was booming and passionate. In three months, the woman encouraged him to live with her and the four children. He told her that it is better not to rush. In less than a month the woman was not picking up his calls, and that was the end of the relationship.

- ▶ Don't think of replacing your ex: God created us with our specific characters and behaviours, hobbies and dreams. There is no one under the sun who is identical in everything. So do not try to replace your ex, because no one is going to be the same as your ex. You have had something special, and that will always be the case. It is important to remember those memories, but finding a new man or a new woman is not about finding a like replacement. This is literarily impossible. If a woman has tension with her ex, the new man should let her handle it. A man can support the woman and encourage her, but he must not contact her ex on her behalf or get involved in an ongoing court battle over their custody agreement. The friend I have quoted in advice number 7 above, informed me the ex-husband of his woman was living some two kilometres away from where the divorced woman and her four children live. He said, "One day I asked the woman to show me the divorce certificate, she promised to show me but never did, until she shut me out."

- ▶ A transitional relationship may help: In Australia, having a transitional relationship is not wrong, it is lawful. If you want to take that path, don't rush into a serious long-term relationship, but start with something less intense. This could be a good way of getting accustomed to seeing a new man or new woman. There is no age limit on having fun in Australia, so take your time to identify the right person. I can recall when I took my mother, aged 90 years, for an X-Ray in Hampton Park, Victoria, and a staff member on duty said to me, "Is this your wife?" At first, I was angry with the staff member, but when I reflected on the statement (there is no age limit on having a relationship in Australia) I then cooled down and said that this is my mother.

▶ When you are in a sugar relationship, don't overdo it: Having multi-relationships can be complicated in your life. Make sure not to make promises you cannot keep, or to lead others on if you are unsure about your own feelings. It is important to be open and honest, and not to find yourself seriously committed to more than one person

▶ Accept that her top priority is always her children: In other relationships, one may have been able to gauge a woman's feelings for him by how much time and energy she puts into the relationship. However, when you are dating a single mother or a widow, this may not necessarily be the case. He may not have the time to see you as often as she'd like, and it is not always easy to hire a baby sitter to allow her to go out. It is also important for a man to know that when he wants to date a single mother with children, he should allow her to handle 100% of the kids' discipline. About 80% of the problems in a family remarriage are caused by children. The new man should never attempt to discipline the children of a single mother and vice versa, to avoid causing problems. The only exception to this rule is if she specifically asks the new man for support or help. When the new man is concerned about the kids' behaviour, he should talk with his new wife privately. A man should never attempt to handle the issue himself without discussing it with her first. Otherwise, this could cause depression and frustration in the man.

▶ Be trustworthy: As a single mother or a widow, the new woman might have experienced situations previously where she depended on a husband who was not trustworthy. As you are going to develop a relationship with her, set yourself apart by being someone she can trust. Be responsible "to her" without being responsible "for her". Although you have a tremendous amount of pressure to provide for her children financially and emotionally, listen to the things she's going through without trying to solve every problem for her. She is strong and she knows how to work it out in time. You can have a successful marriage by listening to what your new wife wants.

▸ Disclose to your partner if you have kids: You must disclose if you are a parent from your first marriage. Being a parent is such an important part of who you are, that you shouldn't hide it. When and how you do it varies by what you feel is right for your own family.

▸ Some people feel that if they disclose that they have kids from the first marriage, this may scare off the potential partner. Don't worry about scaring them off; a potential lover must know that you are a parent. Don't wait too long and worse still, don't lie about how many kids you have. Introduce honesty and trust issues before, so a relationship can blossom. It is recommended that when introducing your new man or woman to your children, it is good to ask yourself these questions:

▸ A woman questions herself first, "Am I ready to be with this man who is not my husband? Will I be happy in our remarriage environment? Will my children be happy with him or will they be sad?"

▸ Similarity a man should ask himself the same questions. It is always advisable for both to also ask their children, especially when they are grown up, "Are you ready to see your mother with a man who is not your father? Will you be happy for me or be sad?"

▸ Respect your time and be as flexible as you can: It is reported that spontaneity is a challenge for single mothers, especially if their kids are younger than high school age. Do your best to schedule outings well ahead of time and be patient if those plans go haywire. Sometimes she may run late because her toddler puked down her top and she has to change, or sometimes visitors may drop into the house unexpectedly and she is to be with them for some hours.

▸ It is generally reported that widowers tend to jump into the dating scene after losing a spouse, long before they are emotionally ready for any kind of relationship. They view the loss of their spouse as a problem that needs to be fixed with a new relationship and for them this is the best way to mend their broken heart.

▶ In contrast, widows tend to wait longer before committing themselves in relationships with other men — but the reality is that some of them don't. Most widows get their lives and hearts in order before testing the water of the new relationship. As a result, they are generally ready for more serious relationships and have fever issues than widowers when looking for new lovers.

▶ Study shows that there are no age differences in widows, that is whether they are in their 30s or 70s; they tend to make same mistakes. In other words, they tend to process grief in a similar manner; they start dating because they want companionship and not a relationship. As a result, many serious relationships of widowers end up in disaster, because they are still grieving.

▶ As we discussed earlier, there is nothing wrong with a man dating soon after losing his spouse, but the best thing he should do is to date a lot of different women to get used to going out with someone other than his late wife. However, he should not latch onto the first woman that shows interest in him. Whenever he finds himself falling for someone, he must take things slowly so that he can decide if he is getting in a relationship for the right reasons. That will save him and the woman he is dating a lot of unnecessary heartache.

▶ It has been reported that when going on a first date, it is common for a man to feel guilty because he would think that he is cheating on his late wife. As a matter of fact, it is hard sometimes for him to concentrate on the date or even hold a conversation with the new woman or with other people around him. Truly speaking, those thoughts and feelings will become less and less on the second date and almost gone by the third date. However, people are different; if those feelings aren't diminishing, he should take a break from dating.

What do children feel about the remarrying of their mother or father?

The question of how children feel about their mother or father remarrying another man or another woman is a huge issue for the majority of widows and widowers in African Australian communities, as well as across the globe. There are many reasons why remarrying has become an issue among the African community. One of the reasons may be that a widow who wants to remarry may have three to four grown up children. Similarly, a man who marries a widow or single mother may also have children. This may cause some problems in the family, although the children may only have a slight acquaintance with their stepfather or stepmother. In a worst-case scenario, the children may not love nor respect the stepfather or stepmother. In this situation it would be good for both stepfather and stepmother to seek support from their community, counsellors or trusted friends as it may help establish a harmonious family relationship.

More importantly, when a person decides to remarry, the two must introduce their prospective spouse to their children as early as possible. Much of any initial negative reaction is because the individuals involved really do not know each other. It is suggested that the new couple should introduce themselves to each other's family after five or six months of the relationship. We hear that some people say that they do not know the right time for introducing themselves to children. Some people wait for two months and others wait for a year, which implies that there is no solid guideline for when to introduce your partner to your children.

Self-introduction is very important to avoid men who are purely seeking out single mothers for whatever reasons. Sophia Benoit (2019) observes that there are no guidelines for how and when one should introduce his/her partner to their children; and there is no guarantee that following this introduction, it will work for your family's situation. Thus, dating as a parent means constantly juggling and negotiating multiple people's needs and wants. There may be tough questions asked by the couples, yet there will be no right answer to the questions. One of these questions could be, "Is it easier to date someone who doesn't have kids?"

One of my informants was telling me that one of the most difficult issues in dating a woman with children is being flexible. Many of women who want to date value flexibility (spontaneity), which is not possible for some men. And the second issue is time management — how to divide one's time to look after the children and one's private affairs; getting everything done on time and well. Some men say they don't have financial resources to pay for babysitters or to pay for childcare. For these reasons, some men are not interested in a relationship with women who have small children.

If it was possible, the couple should have let the children in both families get acquainted before they come together as husband and wife or before they announce their marriage plans. So, once they are comfortable with their decision to marry, they can then make their announcement to their children. Don't put them together in one room when you are announcing your plans for marriage. As you meet them separately and privately, ask for their good will, as most loving children would want remarriage of their mother or father to succeed and they would be supportive. On the other side, the children may not accept a spouse completely, so in this case when meeting the children, one should be natural and friendly as much as possible. A spouse should not try to be what he/she is not. Especially when the children are too young; respect them for who they are. A spouse must be sensitive to the children's grief over the loss of their mother or father. However, back in Africa, it appears children are hardly ever consulted when the mother or the father want to remarry.

Although we are suggesting that a man and a woman should introduce their intention to remarry to their children before they come together, the bottom line is that the ideology of remarriage itself may still be painful to the children. If the children make you uneasy for any major reason, have a serious conversation about your feelings, and don't think that your partner does not like your children. Although the feelings of adult children regarding your remarrying must be considered, the final decision must be made by both of you for the interests of all. Some of your children may be negative towards any relationship you want to enter. They may still be economically and emotionally dependent on you as a parent, and they may feel neglected if you remarry. On the other hand, if your children are opposed to your remarriage because of some specific loving concerns, consider these aspects carefully. While you should be concerned about the feelings of your children, you need to take charge of your life and do what you believe is best, and your remarriage should not cause any separation between you and your children.

The most logical step is to discuss your children's reactions with your trusted relatives and friends or persons who are somewhat detached from your situation. They can best give you objective advice about your relationship.

Absorbing young children into a new marriage may be a major source of conflict for both spouses. The stepfather's or stepmother's role may be demanding and traumatic, when young children are involved. It has been observed by many people that a husband and a wife may agree on nearly everything except how to raise children — their own or someone else's. It is nearly impossible to remain detached from such problems once a couple is united in a remarriage.

Thus, one important thing people intending to remarry should know is that the remarriage will be a major adjustment for adult children, who may not be living with their parents under the same roof or in the same home. For this to be successful, reassure your adult children that you still love them. They should feel welcome to call you and see you, within the bounds of common courtesy and good sense.

Having a new spouse should not cause one to be isolated from their children, even if they have misinformation about the marriage or the new spouse. This can make children hate the new husband or wife. It is commonly believed that playing "mind games" with each other's children is a sure way of breeding major problems in a marriage. When a couple has problems in the house, they should try to resolve it themselves.

Often the family situation is still more challenging when you remarry a divorced person and bring a child or children who have been living with the ex-spouse into your new home. Some children of divorced parents are very troublesome. Some of them, when they grow up, even want to fight their stepfather, but very few children who are brought from the father's side want to fight their stepmother. They have a great capacity to spread rumours wherever they go. Therefore, both the man and woman who want to remarry must think about this very seriously before making their decision for remarrying. Don't let the present grief of your mate's death cause you to enter a new marriage that is risky for all involved. Of all the issues that may come up in remarriage in Australia, it is the problem of social security (Centrelink money) and wages that each may earn which can be the deadliest and may even force partners to divorce again.

Are you sexually compatible?

One of the most important aspects of any marriage is the degree of sexual satisfaction attained by each of the partners. We should understand that a person's need for sexual gratification cannot be terminated at the death of a mate. There is a lot of research data which shows that most healthy persons remain sexually active up to the age of 80 years and beyond.

If you intend to remarry, discuss your degree of sexual interest in this area with your prospective mate as it has been disclosed that most Africans like to test their sexual interest in bed before re-marrying. There is potential for a great amount of stress during sex. Experiences from community members say that if a person who has previously had an active sex life and is marrying someone who has little interest in sexual intimacy, this means they are marrying a 'walking- dead person'. Therefore, testing in bed is of paramount importance. The same is true if they have different ideas of how to express that intimacy. One of my informants told me that his woman is not always ready for sex whenever they are in bed. She keeps on pushing him away and telling him to wait because she is not yet ready. The man said, "I thought when we are together in the bedroom, she would be ready for sex within 30 minutes, unfortunately this is not the case."

Many women who are experiencing sexual arousal difficulties rarely discuss the issue with their doctor or gynaecologist. When women visit their gynaecologist, they usually ask, "Am I sexually active? Can I have birth control?" But they rarely tell the gynaecologist whether they are really enjoying sex life. The stigma surrounding women and sex, especially good sex, runs so deep in women that the very idea of what it means to have good sex is murky, filtered by unrealistic portrayals of women on screen. Their orgasm usually comes seductively after five seconds of penetration. Sexual pressure lights up their brains, essentially flooding it with oxygen. Study shows that more oxygen to the brain boosts cognitive function, so higher levels of sexual activity can help protect one's cognitive functioning.

Body image sometimes also puts pressure on women because they want to look a certain way, to be of a certain weight, or this is how they should feel, instead of thinking about having good sex. A woman can talk positively all the time about what she likes, but nothing would make her feel great about her own body. She may watch or hear of people with an aspirational body type getting turned on by each other, desiring each other, and having an amazing time in bed with their partners.

Having discussed "enjoyment of sex life in women" let us now try to answer the question "How does a woman own her pleasure?" Different people may give different answers to this question, but the reality is that if a woman wants to own her pleasure, the first thing she can do is to get behind the idea that her sexual pleasure should be prioritized. It is reported that from the moment a woman is born, she is brought up to believe that she has to be selfless to everybody around her in a way a man isn't. But when a woman becomes self-ish and enjoys herself, this may affect some men.

In the twenty-first century, a woman deserves to focus on herself without outside interference. She needs to talk about pleasure until the uncomfortable silences in her mind disappear. Therefore, today we see many women talk openly about female pleasure and their relationship to it. One writer called Eckert, says, "Relationships win, communication wins, and women win because there's freedom to speak about things that have otherwise been stigmatized or taboo." With these views in mind, I would like to suggest to both men and women that your "motto" is to "own your sexual health and your sexual pleasure because these are your power".

Many women do not know how to relieve stress and improve their sleep. It is healthy to have masturbation as it is a safe and natural way to feel good; discover what gets you hot, and release built-up sexual tension. Masturbation is a safe way to release sexual tension during pregnancy, however, masturbation may not be safe for women in a high-risk pregnancy. This is because orgasm can increase a woman's chances of going into labour. Some people may develop an addiction to masturbation, and this can harm a relationship as well as some parts of life. Masturbation does not have any harmful side effect, although some women may feel guilty of being addicted to it. Some may feel guilty of masturbation because of cultural, spiritual beliefs. There is nothing wrong with masturbation or immoral, but we still hear messages from religious leaders that masturbation is dirty and shameful.

What will your living arrangements be?

For the new couple to make a genuine and reasonable living arrangement, they should first answer the following questions before deciding to remarry. These questions include, but are not limited to:

- ▶ Will you live in the other person's home or in your own home?
- ▶ Will you both sell your houses (if you have one) or will you buy or rent a new dwelling place that is jointly yours?
- ▶ Will you have his or her children and your own children live together with you?
- ▶ Will you use some of each other's furniture or buy everything new?
- ▶ How will you dispose of items not needed in the new home?

Experience and survey data in Australia show that there are no clear-cut answers for the above important questions, but if African Australians use their traditional minds, they will have simple answers to those questions. The traditional answer is, "When a man and a woman remarry, a wife must move with her children and some of her good furniture into the home of the new man. The remaining furniture can be left behind for relatives or older children. The new husband is expected to have enough new furniture to start off. She can bring along children of school age, the older children can be left behind with an uncle or aunty."

However, African Australians need to judge each situation individually because people are not the same. For this reason, it is important for the new couple to find a plan that will satisfy both. Culturally, African men when they get remarried or married, they do not move to live in the woman's home, rather a woman comes and lives in the man's home. But in Australia, most African Australians don't live in their own properties, they rent these properties. So, when renting a house, the couple must decide on whether to live in the other's house or to rent a new house. But the best option is for the couple to live in man's house rather than living in the woman's house even although this property is being rented. This is simply to bring the feeling, for especially a woman, that I am now married in my husband's house.

Avoid comparison of your deceased with the new mate

Science tells us that every human being has their own character, and when you want to remarry after the death of your husband or your wife, don't think that you will find a mate exactly like your first one. Your new husband or wife will have some good and bad sides your first mate did not have. For more information about the good and bad sides of a man or a woman, please see chapter 10.

Remarrying can be good or bad depending on how you prepare yourself, but when you want to prepare for remarriage, you should not place your former mate on a pedestal and challenge your new partner to be the same. No, this cannot work. Similarly, leaving the photo of the deceased spouse on the wall and from time to time remarking that your former partner "was so good" about doing such and such things, is not conducive to a harmonious second marriage. Conversely, it is not good to expose all the faults of your former spouse to your new spouse. Be fair and objective about your first mate, without making direct or indirect comparisons. One thing a person should not forget is that what happened in one's first marriage can repeat itself in the second marriage.

Should you have a prenuptial agreement and a new Will?

In African culture, a Will or prenuptial agreement is not important because there are traditional laws that guide the survivor and relatives of the deceased on what to do when someone dies. The only things a dying African can tell his or her close relatives before their last breath may include if he/she is owed some money from someone that needs to be paid, or if he/she owes money to someone; if he/she has something in their heart that might be disturbing them at this last moment; requesting the brothers to look after any children — this only in the case of a man; and calling the children to live in unity and harmony.

Being in a new social environment like Australia makes Africans think outside the box. As a result, the majority of Africans in Australia believe that it is important for a couple, who want to remarry, to establish a prenuptial agreement and a new Will before their second marriage. The research I have conducted among Africans revealed that some of African Australians are now making a new prenuptial agreement and a new Will. This is especially true where children are involved and if either of partners have various financial holdings. In the event of the first or second divorce or death of one spouse, each mate needs to have a clear understanding of his or her legal rights. The research also revealed that some of the Africans get remarried without making a new prenuptial agreement and new Will for the fear of potential divorce.

Interestingly in Australia, this responsibility is taken on by lawyers or a Will Officer where the deceased will leave his/her Will. This helps avoid unnecessary quarrels among children of the deceased. Therefore, the new Wills for the remarrying couple are absolutely a must, so that each of the family members will receive their entitlement or portion. The new couple should also make sure they formalise their wishes regarding any other separate or joint heirs. They must be sure it is mentioned within their Will that a prenuptial agreement has been made. If it is not mentioned in the Will, there can be considerable heartache for all concerned. To do this correctly, the couple must look for local lawyers who specialize in premarital agreements and Wills.

Traditionally, before a person dies, that person is asked whether she/he has some money in the bank or in debts (loans). This can offer an opportunity for the person to tell people what should be done with the money or where to collect debts when she/he dies. Soon after the death of a spouse, the relatives of the deceased husband (not of the wife) take responsibility for implementing the orders made by the dead spouse.

Why men choose one woman over another?

It was reported that a woman was looking at her ex's new girlfriend and wondering what he found in her. The new girlfriend was not even smarter or funnier than her, but the man still chose the new girlfriend over her. She couldn't stop thinking, why is this?

It is unfortunate that in this world some people think that love is mysterious where two people are attracted to each other by destiny. Thus, in real life we should understand there are some important factors which make a person fall in love with another person and they stay with that person for life. Therefore, some women who may be in a same situation of the lady described above, should not continue asking themselves repeatedly what is wrong with them. If you are one of those women who continue asking themselves, "Why our men have chosen a new woman over us", the following seven points may help you to answer the question.

> ► They have the same family values:

During your relationship, you might not have the same goal as your ex. For example, your ex's main goal of a relationship was to settle down. Now he has found a woman who shares the same family values and she has the same plans. This means that your goal was completely different; you do not want to marry and have children, but he wants marriage and children right now. Therefore, instead of waiting for you to change your mind, he thinks it's easier to find someone else who has the same family values.

When he finds a perfect match and true soul mate, he would not look any further. Although sometimes a man may think it is hard to decide who is the one for him, but there are some common traits that will always ring true with the heart. When a man is faced with the question "Who is the one for me?" this man should not worry, because time will tell him. Once he finds her, he does not need to worry or look for women any further, because that true love in him is a magical thing and it identifies itself before his eyes. It becomes something he cannot even use words to describe.

How can a person know that she/he has finally found the one they are truly looking for? Study shows that there are five signs that can show a person that they have found the true beloved one. These signs include: -

- ▸ You truly can't imagine your life without that person: True harmony is when you find a perfect person you know and believe that you cannot be who you are without her/him. At this stage, you feel complete and you don't want to go around without that person. Each person enjoys how much time she/he has with that person.

- ▸ You have developed a partnership that balances both of you perfectly: This means the relationship just works and the two of you feel that you have found a good partnership together. However, you may play different roles at different times, yet you are in harmony together. You have found a way of making things work both for you.

- ▸ You can see a future together: If you want to make plans for your future, take vacations and spend free time together to go through what you want for your life in the short and long term. This means you see a future together and let each one play active roles in building your life.

- ▸ You can overlook the little things for the big picture: This means that everything in a person you love is perfect but don't dwell much on the small things, it's better that you focus on the big picture; the little things can spoil your life. Don't get irritated if your partner has done something quirky, for example chewing gum during your meeting, rather learn how to embrace one another. If you come across some odd habits in your partner, it's better to let them pass with ease.

- You cannot feel pure happiness being with someone else other than your beloved one: Both of you may be undoubtedly happy. You are quite contented with each other and want to make things work for both of you. If this is the case, you can say with certainty that you have found your best match because all things that you want in a person are present. You can now conclude in your heart that this is the one and only one that you need in your life.

- **He loves her confidence:**

- You might have been unsure about your relationship and he has obviously noticed it. Don't forget that men are also seeking confidence and reliability in a relationship, just as women do. This implies that when a man finds someone who can provide it for him, it's more likely that he will choose this person over you. Every woman, who is seeking a genuine and lasting relationship, should understand that it is great to share everything with her man, but when a woman tells him about her insecurities, his confidence with her would disappear as well. This is the second reason why your man may decide to choose a new woman over you.

- **They have better sex:**

- Sex life is very important in the relationship of any healthy couple. Culturally, it is believed that when a man has fallen in love with a woman, and before the declaration of the marriage, both must have sexual intercourse as many times as they can. If during these meetings, a man finds that the woman meets all sexual criteria better than his other partner, he would then feel more attracted to this woman than to his other partner.

- Having better sex is one of the factors that attracts a man to a woman. However, we should understand that sex is not the only attractive factor, there are other factors. Of course, if the only reason why a man has chosen the new woman is sex, this means their romance won't last long. A good relationship needs other ingredients. When these ingredients are around, their bond will become even stronger, if they are compatible in this intimate part of life. This is the third reason why your man may decide to choose a new woman over you.

- **She never pressured him:**
- It is generally believed that when it comes to relationships, most men feel pressured and obliged to commit to their partners, especially when a woman starts to question all the man's decisions and particularly his feelings. No wonder, in such a situation, a man would choose whoever does not look down on him 24 hours, seven days a week. A woman without much pressure is more desirable to most men.
- Treat your sugar daddy with respect always and be compassionate, don't treat him like an "ATM". Build trust with your sugar daddy, don't be a scammer. Being honest is always the key in every situation. Yes, you are there for money and gifts and all that you want, but you don't have to be all about money, because he is there to help you, himself and also family members when it applies.
- To earn your sugar daddy's respect, you must be honest about what you want and who you are. Your personality is what make you attractive; don't make your man feel like he is developing a relationship with a person who doesn't care enough how he maintains his life and the lives of his other dependants. If you want to respect your man, you should have disciplined manners because earning respect starts with respecting oneself — set straightforward boundaries and follow through, so don't pick a man just because of hunger for money. This is the fourth reason why your man may decide to choose a new woman over you.
- **They share the same interests:**
- One of the mistakes some women make is that they fail to understand that "sharing the same interests is a powerful bond between men and

women". It is true that a man can love a woman because she is beautiful, smart and funny, but it's never the same as when he is with a woman who also likes the same song and plays his private computer games. The two may also have the same cultural values, which is all about their personalities, and one can do nothing to change it. This is the fifth reason why your man may decide to choose a new woman over you.

- ▶ **His friends and family members love her:**
- ▶ Choice of a woman in Africa cultures is sometimes influenced by what the lover's friends and family members have on the woman. The more a woman is loved by the majority of a man's friends and family members, the more likely the man would choose that woman. Thus, many times a man chooses one woman over the other because she is loved by his friends and family members who may love her more than you. Therefore, the opinions of close relatives and best friends influence the decision of the man looking for a woman. Some women do not like the way some men are shaped by opinions of their relatives or friends, but they can do nothing to change this.
- ▶ Experiences show that when the mother of the man prefers the other woman over the other, the man will likely listen to his mother, because the man would not like to build a wall between him and relatives as well as trusted friends. Family co-existence is very important in African culture; no one can play with it. This is the sixth reason why your man may decide to choose a new woman over you.
- ▶ **She is independent:**
- ▶ Some of the women in African society do not like to depend on men (especially those who are now in diaspora), they are more independent. So, one of the reasons why a man chooses a woman over another is because she is not depending on him for everything — although she may indirectly be but she does not show it. Most of men around the globe like women who are free and not dependent on them for every small thing. This implies that if a woman in love stops looking after

herself and puts more pressure on a man to support her, their relationship will not last long. Most men who choose women to settle
down, would look for someone who talks the talk and walks the walk.
Of course, there are some men who may want to decide everything in
relationship, but the reality is that the majority of men would prefer
someone who can think and do things independently. You can't expect
someone to be with you if you don't satisfy each other on certain level.
This is the seven reason why your man may decide to choose a new
woman over you.

Chapter Seven
Sex After Birth

Menstrual Cycle

Before a woman gives birth to a baby, she needs to go through some processes that include menstrual cycle and conception or pregnancy. The menstrual cycle is the monthly series of changes a woman's body goes through in the preparation for the possibility of a pregnancy. Each month, one of the ovaries releases an egg — this process is known as ovulation. At this time, hormonal changes prepare the uterus for pregnancy. Ovaries release an egg between the 11th and 18th day following the first day of menstrual cycle; and this is the time a woman is most likely to get pregnant. But some African women believe that the dangerous period for a woman to get pregnant is the first day following the shedding of the blood. This is not true, because science tells us that if ovulation takes place and the egg is not fertilized, the lining of the uterus sheds through the vagina. This process is known as menstrual period.

The menstrual period which is counted from the first day of one period to the first day of the next menstruation is different for every woman. Menstrual flow may occur every 21 to 35 days and last between two and seven days or more. The menstrual cycle may be regular, which could last about the same time every month or somewhat irregular. The period of a woman may be heavy or light, painful or painless, long or short and still be considered normal. Within a broad range, normal is what is normal for a woman. (Dr Len Kliman, 2020).

A woman should consult her doctor should she find that her periods suddenly stop for more than ninety days and she is not pregnant.

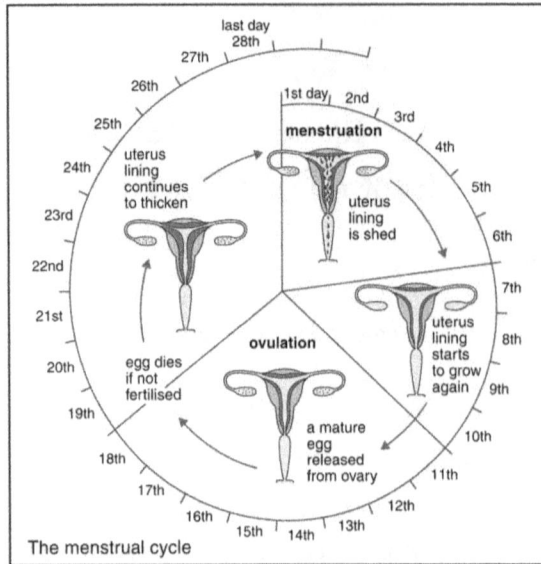

Figure: 30. Menstrual cycle

Childbirth

Giving birth is no easy feat, no matter what kind of labour a woman may have. It can translate into physical symptoms, including sores and dryness during sex.

It is always better for a woman to listen to her body when re-exploring her sex life again. More importantly, if a woman has a tear during a birth delivery, it is best to keep an eye on how it is healing, before thinking about having sex. Women tend to assume that after their bodies have bounced back from childbirth, their sex lives should do the same. A lot of women soon come to realise that sex after birth simply does not feel the same. Sometimes a woman may not have sexual desire. (Pamela Levin MD, (2015).

We know that sexual desire is very important for relationships and sexual satisfaction. A study that focused on couples found that the more people experienced sexual desire throughout the day, the better their sex lives were. For this reason, it is advisable for men and women not to switch off sexual desires during the day, because this could lead them to a better time in bedroom.

In human beings, sex desire changes from moment to moment. Research showed that the when-and-how a person experiences sexual desire varies from person to person. Some people think that men have a stronger sexual desire than women, but the reality is this is not true. The fact is that scientists found that men think more about sex than women, they think about sex 34 times in a day (that is about every 1,700 seconds) and women about 19 times a day.

There is no right and wrong time to start having sex again after childbirth. However, a woman should not rush into it, because if sex hurts, it won't be pleasurable. It is not unusual for a woman to feel less like having sex than she used to, because she may feel tired. A woman should also not forget to apply family planning, as it is possible for her to get pregnant again three weeks after giving birth. For this reason, women are advised to wait around 2-4 weeks before starting intercourse, this is roughly the time bleeding is also expected to stop. Otherwise, they will be in high risk of haemorrhage and infection. (Elizabeth Atkin, 2019).

Dr Sandra Wheatley (2019) observes that the best time to have sex again is when a woman feels like it, three months is the average, but it can also take up to a year or two to feel comfortable physically and emotionally. The reality is that everyone is different, and some mothers have confessed that they have had sex four months after birth, while others confessed that they have had sex one day after birth.

Having sex one day after childbirth may not be wise, for example, when a woman has a C-section during childbirth she may need to wait a little longer. And for a woman who has had a tear or episiotomy and stitches, she is required to wait until her six weeks' check-up by her family doctor. Many women found sex uncomfortable after their caesarean, but eventually they will manage to get back into the swing of things.

Therefore, when a woman is not ready for sex, she should not feel shy about telling her partner the problem—tension will make things worse. It is important for a woman to listen to her body, as every woman's journey is different.

Can the vagina change after childbirth?

It is natural for every woman to have her vagina change after childbirth and it might even feel wider, dry or sore for some days. Dr Suzy Elneil (2018) a consultant in urogynaecology at University College Hospital, London says, "The vagina can feel looser, softer and more open after birth. It may also look and feel bruised or swollen." This is normal and swelling and openness should start to reduce a few days after baby's birth. However, it may not return completely to its pre-birth shape, but this is not a problem and a woman should not worry about it.

It is important to know that when a woman gives birth, the baby travels through the cervix and out through the vagina, which is also called "birth canal". The entrance to the vagina always stretches to allow the baby through. Sometimes the baby may find it difficult to get through the vagina; in this case the doctor or midwife may cut the skin between the vagina and anus (known as perineum, see figure 15) to allow the baby out. This action, in medical terms, is known as an "episiotomy". Pamela Levin MD (2015) observes that women who have had an episiotomy or who experienced a tear during birth may find sex painful for the first few months after childbirth. A woman's relationship with a partner might also change after childbirth. As such during this transitional period, a woman's interest in sex may not match up with her partner's interest for sex. Most of our African Australians do not know if they can talk to their doctors about challenges with their sex lives, so I want to encourage them to do so.

Although the vagina area may feel painful or sore after birth, the good news is that it usually improves within 6-12 weeks after the birth. Pelvic floor exercises always help the situation. It is important to keep the perineal area (see figure 15) clean every day by having a bath or shower. Pelvic floor exercises can be done anywhere and at any time; a woman can do this while sitting or standing up by doing the following:

- Squeeze and draw in your anus, at the same time close up and draw your vagina upwards.
- Do it quickly, tightening and releasing the muscles immediately.
- Then do it slowly, holding the contractions for as long as you can, but no more than 10 seconds before you relax.
- Repeat each exercise ten times, for about four to six times a day.
- Source: Dr Suzy Elneil, 2028, PP. 1-4).

Can a woman still have an orgasm after giving birth?

The answer to this question is simple and clear, researchers found that a woman can still have orgasms after giving birth, however it may take a bit longer to get there. The most important thing is that a woman should take it easy, and rather focus on having fun in other ways and enjoying her partner. It is natural for a woman's libido to change after giving birth. Some women may find their libido higher than usual; others may find the opposite. Dr Wheatley suggests, "The real relationship killer is loss of intimacy, keep your intimacy by having some skin to skin with your partner, let your partner give you a relaxing massage. As I keep on mentioning in this book that although sex is important, it's more than a physical act but it is an emotional connection. Plus, it releases hormones that bond a man and a woman together.

Reasons why a woman may struggle to have an orgasm after giving birth

Many researchers have found that the months after childbirth are the most vulnerable ones of a woman's life. Her hormones are running rampant, leaving her more emotional than ever, and her body is trying to recover from giving birth. One thing a woman realises at this time is that she may have trouble orgasming after birth. However, this is not uncommon, but a woman may still wonder why she is struggling to achieve an orgasm.

According to Maggie May Ethride (2016) women are struggling to achieve postpartum orgasms after giving birth because of the following five reasons: -

▶ Because a woman was torn during childbirth: When a baby comes out of the vagina of a woman, we say "her body rips". This often requires some post-delivery stitching and healing, which can make a woman hesitant to have sex. Even if a woman does have sex, it might not be as good since the nerve connections have not fully recovered yet. Therefore, it is better for a woman to give her body time to heal and she will find that orgasms will return in no time.

▶ Because a woman has a low libido: Medical professionals note that it is normal to have a reduced sex drive months after labour, and there are many reasons for this. Fatigue from looking after the baby or the stress from a new financial situation can make a woman not in the mood for sex. This won't last forever. It was found by Henrietta Hughes, a general practitioner in London, that many mothers experience a significant decrease in tiredness, an improvement in mood, and an increase in sexual activity, sexual feelings and frequency of sex within four weeks of stopping breastfeeding.

▶ A woman may have pelvic floor issues: The pelvic floor plays an important role in sexual function, as it contracts during sex and orgasm, creating pleasurable sensations. Medically, a woman's pelvic floor is a group of muscles located in her pelvis which stretch like a hammock from the pubic bone (at the front) to the coccyx or tail bone (at the back) and from side to side. These muscles are stretched during childbirth, and while they do bounce back, sometimes they need a little help. A woman should do pelvic floor exercises, which can assist in toning up those muscles, getting her back to normal.

▶ A woman may have post-partum depression: Some women think of the enormous physical and hormonal changes that she is going through following the delivering of a baby, and this often leads to postpartum depression (PPD). Mental Health America estimates that twenty percent of new mothers experience post-partum depression, which can result in a huge loss of sex drive and ability to orgasm. A woman should treat her PPD and return to a normal state of orgasm soon.

▶ A woman may have vagina dryness: Healthline reports that post-pregnancy hormonal changes after childbirth, which usually results in the vaginal dryness, makes intercourse painful and orgasms difficult to achieve. Thus, when a woman is experiencing vaginal dryness, she should use a natural based vaginal lubrication, and this can help her achieve orgasm. (Pamela Levin MD, 2015).

Chapter Eight
Menopause

What is menopause?

"While menopause is natural and normal, husbands and wives are often caught off-guard by changes in their marriage relationship. Many husbands become confused by the behaviour of their wives in menopause." By David Hager (2018)

Menopause is a natural decline in reproductive hormones in a woman. However, there are many definitions of "menopause". For the purpose of this book, we are going to define menopause as *"time in a woman's life, when her period has stopped for twelve consecutive months; and it marks the end of fertility. She can no longer become pregnant naturally"*. Dr Nicola Gates (2019) says, "Count twelve months of no period and you can claim you are in menopause, unless you have had a hysterectomy." (P. 69).

According to David Hager (2018) menopause is the point in life when a woman's ovaries get smaller and stop producing the hormones called oestrogen, progesterone and testosterone". Oestrogen and progesterone are the hormones that control the menstrual cycle, the production of eggs is depleted and fertility declines. Dr Nicola Gates (2019) observes that with menopause, the functions of oestrogen and progesterone have ceased, and a woman's body is adjusting to lower levels of less potent oestrogen. But the woman is still having oestrogen to maintain her health, although now she relies on a different form made in different places in her body and the oestrogen is now in much lower quantities than before. The woman's body at this stage relies on oestrogen in the same way as a man's body. Oestrogen also influences memory and the brain structures associated with memory. Therefore, low levels of oestrogen mean low levels of specific neurotransmitters required for memory formation, which reduces the amount of information transfer and consolidation. Menopause is a healthy and normal part of women's lives, shifting their bodies from cycling hormones for fertility to hormone stability for health maintenance. Unless it is a medical or surgical menopause, it takes time, with most women experiencing changes in their bodies, before their periods finally ease. (PP. 69-70, 132). Oestrogen affects many parts of the body, which include blood vessels, heart, bone, breast, uterus, urinary system, skin, and brain. Loss of oestrogen is believed to be the cause of many of the symptoms associated with menopause. At the time of menopause, the ovaries also decrease their production of testosterone, this is a hormone involved with sex drive. (Traci C. Johnson, MD, 2018). According to Nicola Gates (2019), menopause is caused by the reduction of oestrogen and progesterone in a woman's body, leaving the body to adjust to lower levels of less potent oestrogen (as we have discussed above). The changes and symptoms women experience during the transition are due to the loss of the super-charged source of oestrogen. Sometimes there may be so many other things going on in life that the absence of periods is not even noticed (PP. 69-70).

Menopause occurs naturally when a woman's ovaries run out of functioning eggs. At the time of birth, most females have about 1 to 3 million eggs, which are gradually lost throughout a woman's life. By the time of a girl's first menstrual period, she has an average of about 400,000 eggs and by the time of menopause, a woman may have fewer than 10,000 eggs. A small percentage of these eggs are lost through normal ovulation and most eggs die off through a process called "atresia".

It is important to note that menopause can come with discomfort and inconvenience, but it is not a disease or abnormality. It is a natural time in a woman's life, as we have just mentioned above, and most of the things a woman experiences at the time are typical. Nicola Gates (2019) notes, that most women do not talk about their menopause experiences, either to their partners, friends or family members. For example, when women have hot flushes that could last up to an hour, they never tell other people that they are experiencing hot flushes. This lack of disclosure may threaten relationship satisfaction. (Nicola Gates, 2019).

Some studies reported that about 1% of women around the world begin to develop menopause between the age of 40 to 45 years. When this happen, it is known as premature menopause. Stephanie Watson et al (2019) observes that premature menopause occurs before the age of 40, while the majority of women in the world begin to develop menopause between the age of 45 to 55. According to health workers, there are three stages in menopause, and these are: *Before-During-After.* Rebecca Ashkenazy MD (2019) and Dr Nicola Gates (2019) argue that there are three phases in menopause: Perimenopause, menopause and Post-menopause. The common term used by health workers/professionals is the collective term "Menopause transition". The three stages of menopause are as follows: -

Perimenopause (Before)
This is a period of eight to ten years before a woman's last menstrual cycle. On average, perimenopause may last between three to four years, but in some women, it may last only for a few months. During this transition period, the ovaries of a woman will produce less oestrogen over time. However, she will continue to have menstrual cycles, but the cycles may be irregular and there could still be chance for her to get pregnant.

Menopause (During)
This is a period which confirms that a woman has not had her period for twelve consecutive months.

Post menopause (After)
This is a period after menopause, where a woman's menopause symptoms

may begin to ease; yet she might be at risk for certain conditions such as heart disease to increase. Dr Nicola Gates (2019) observes that women are now increasingly taking ownership of the term "post menopause" to describe the time when they have no more symptoms of menopause and are focusing on the positive liberating aspects of hormone stability (P, 62). As we have discussed before, menopause usually occurs when there has been a change in a woman's reproductive hormones and the ovaries run out of eggs. This can happen naturally and at the expected age or prematurely, as we shall discuss below.

As previously mentioned, the expected age for natural menopause around the world is between 45 -55 years. However, the average expected age for menopause in Australia is between 51-52 years, while in America the expected age is 51 years, though it may occur on average up to 2 years earlier for African American and Latina women. (Jennifer Huizen, 2019).

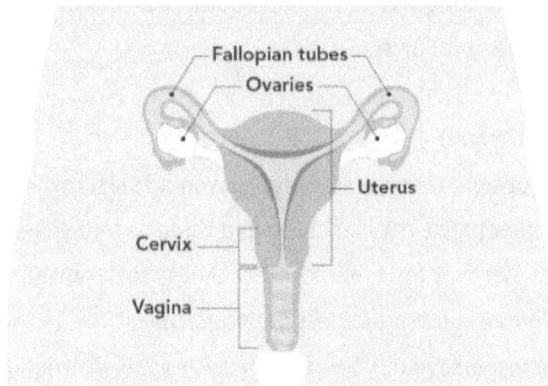

Figure: 31. Pictures of a Natural Ovary

It is considered a natural event when the ovaries instead of continuing with regular periods, they just stop; it can develop more painful periods and as a result, a woman experiences premenstrual syndrome (PMS). Study shows that approximately 20% of women around the world will have no symptoms of menopause. (Jennifer Huizen, 2019).

There are many unknown causes of menopause. Sometimes periods stop spontaneously, and this is referred to as "primary ovarian insufficient" (POI). Several blood tests are usually performed to confirm the POI and to try to find the cause. Therefore, it is recommended that women with POI should undergo hormone therapy. The type of hormone therapy recommended is known as "high-dose" menopausal hormone therapy (MHT)

Menopause can also be caused by surgery (removal of ovaries). This occurs when a woman is still having periods and surgery is performed to remove both ovaries (oophorectomy). We are informed by scientists that the three female hormones, that is, oestrogen, progesterone and testosterone are all released from the ovaries. Therefore, once the ovaries are removed, the levels of oestrogen and testosterone in a woman's body will fall by 50% within 24 hours of the surgery, and this can result in severe menopausal symptoms that interfere with the daily life of a woman. But other reports indicate that some of the symptoms may start within 48 hours of surgery, while others can develop later. (Jennifer Huizen, 2019).

Two ovaries are removed from a woman when she has severe endometriosis which is causing chronic pelvic pain. The pain is chronic because of pelvic inflammatory disease (PID) that involves an infection of the uterus, fallopian tubes or ovaries. The two ovaries can also be removed when a woman has ovarian cancer. So if the two ovaries are not removed a woman will be in high risk of developing breast or ovarian cancer. It is reported that in some women whose ovaries are removed, this may be due to a strong family history of breast or ovarian cancer or due to the presence of certain genetic variants (BRCA-1 or 2) that identify a woman as having this higher risk.

What are the signs and symptoms of menopause?

It appears some women are not aware of the signs and symptoms of menopause, as a result they are often caught off guard and become confused by sudden body changes. Dr Nicola Gates (2019) notes that women often don't talk about periods, which can make it hard to know if they are experiencing normal periods or perimenopausal changes, or the symptoms of something more serious.

It is very easy to think that they have a natural cycle. It is also very common for women to tolerate heavy periods and do nothing about them. Most women can easily recognize changes within themselves as they know their body, its signs and patterns best. But for the health professionals recognising perimenopause is not an easy task as they cannot see what is going on. (P. 64).

Menopause Symptoms

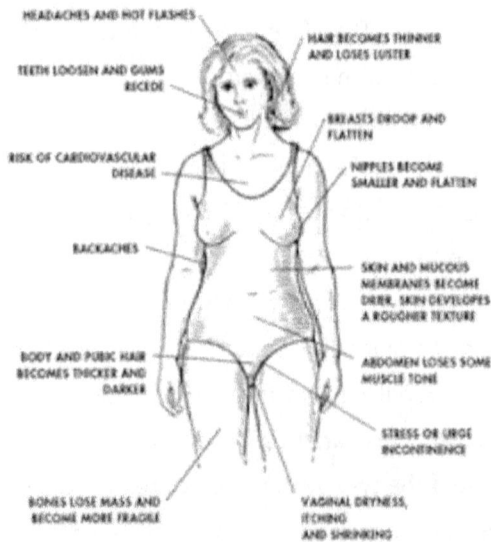

Figure: 32. Menopause Symptoms

Rebecca Ashkenazy, MD, (2019) observes that as a woman approaches menopause, her ovaries make a different number of hormones called oestrogen and progesterone. She may have irregular periods and may also start to have a variety of other menopause signs, which include: -

- ► Hot Flushes, which cause a sudden feeling of heat in the face, neck, chest, back and arms; this can last between a few seconds to ten minutes. A woman may sweat during a hot flush and have cold chills afterwards.

▸ Trouble sleeping,

▸ Vaginal dryness, which can cause itching, burning and discomfort. It may lead to painful intercourse and cuts and tears in the vagina.

▸ Mood swings or irritability

Having examined the signs and symptoms of menopause, it is important for us to note that these symptoms may be different for each woman. It is reported that hot flushes in some women may be severe and may interfere with their lives, while in other women it may be mild. More importantly, some women don't experience any hot flushes at all.

Signs and Symptoms of Early Menopause

Apart from women's ovaries changing and hormone production during the menopause transition, there are multiple changes going on in the body. Ageing is important, as aside from menopause, midlife has its own health changes, with poor health and lifestyle choices also starting to affect the body as women age. Dr Nicola Gates (2019) pointed out that perimenopause often creeps up on women, as they can be unaware of hormonal changes until the cycling levels of oestrogen and progesterone become desynchronised and they experience symptoms. Often the first symptoms of the transition women notice is a change to their menstrual cycle or quality of their periods which may become shorter, longer, heavier, lighter, closer together, further apart, and generally irregular.

Menopause can cause uncomfortable symptoms, such as:

▸ Hot Flushes — Hot flushes are a feeling of intense heat, not caused by external sources, and which can appear suddenly. It is reported that hot flushes are symptoms of menopausal transition and are experience by about 75% of women. The cause of hot flushes remains a mystery, but the best explanation is that the fluctuation and reduction of oestrogen upsets the brain's regulation of body temperature. (Dr Nicola Gates, 2019, P. 85).

▸ Heavy bleeding or lighter periods than one normally experiences.

- Spotting
- Periods that last longer than a week
- Longer amount of time in between periods
- Mood swings
- Changes in sexual feelings or desire
- Vagina dryness
- Trouble sleeping
- Night sweats — when hot flushes occur at night, they are called "night sweats" and they ruin women's sleep.
- Loss of bladder control
- Less frequent menstruation
- Weight gain
- Depression
- Anxiety
- Difficulty concentrating
- Memory problems
- Reduced orgasm and sex drive in women — new research suggests that the size and shape of one's face may predict sex drive, attitudes to casual sex, and even likelihood to cheat
- Dry skin
- Increased urination
- Sore or tender breasts
- Headaches
- Reduced muscle mass
- Painful or stiff joints
- Reduced bone mass
- Less full breasts
- Hair thinning or loss
- Increased hair growth on other areas of the body, such as the face, neck, chest, and upper back.

Having said this, it is important to understand that most women first begin developing menopause symptoms about 4 years before their last period. Only a small number of women experience menopause symptoms for up to a decade before menopause occurs; and 1 in 10 women experience menopause symptoms for 12 years following their last period. (Jennifer Huizen, 2019).

What causes early menopause?

Studies show that causes of early menopause are many, although sometimes the causes can't be determined. According to Stephanie Watson et al (2019) early menopause sometimes is caused when ovaries are damaged. This includes chemotherapy for cancer or an oophorectomy — that is removal of ovaries. Dr Nicola Gates (2019) observes that medical intervention such as treatment for ovarian cancer, or as a preventative measure to reduce breast cancer risk, can cause early or premature menopause. It may involve surgical removal of the ovaries or drug treatment to stop the ovaries from functioning. Chemotherapy or pelvic radiation treatment for cancer may also reduce fertility and cause early menopause, as it may damage the ovaries.

It is good for women to know their menstrual cycle because it provides helpful information regarding their health as well as the function of their ovaries, fertility and general health. It appears that there are many things that can disrupt women's menstrual cycle and stop their ovaries from working before the age of natural menopause. A disruption of the menstrual cycle before real menopause is a serious issue because of its impact upon fertility and health.

When women are in their early twenties, they have their highest fertility, but as they age the fertility starts to get lower and lower. The chance of pregnancy reduces by mid-thirties, as egg quality and quantity are reduced, which lowers fertility, and this is one reason why some women in this age group have issues of becoming pregnant. By age forty, the chance of conception per cycle is as low as 5%, and some women may even be in perimenopause without knowing it. (PP 75-76).

Generally, it is believed that the following four things are the main causes of early or premature menopause: -

- Genetics — where there is no reason for early menopause, we can say it is likely genetic, which means a woman has inherited early menopause from a family member (mostly the mother). Study shows that if a woman's mother started menopause early, the women is more likely to do the same.

- Therefore, it is advisable for a woman, who knows that her mother started menopause early, to discuss genetic testing options with her General Practitioner (GP). Dr Nicola Gates (2019) notes that the cause of naturally occurring premature menopause, as opposed to medical, remains a mystery in most cases. The loss of periods may be a symptom of a bigger health condition or genetic issue such as Fragile X Syndrome and Turner Syndrome, which can cause follicle depletion. (P. 76).

- Chromosome defects: Some chromosome defects can lead to early menopause. A chromosome defect can be detected in a woman when her ovaries don't function properly, and this causes her to enter premature menopause. Other chromosomal defects such as pure gonadal dysgenesis — a variant of Turner Syndrome can also cause early menopause.

- Lifestyle: A study conducted in 2012 about smoking revealed that long-term or regular smokers are likely to experience premature menopause. It is reported that women who smoke may start menopause one or two years earlier that women who don't smoke.

- Thin body: Research shows that oestrogen is stored in fat tissue. This means that women who have a thin body have fewer oestrogen stores, as a result they are more likely to have early menopause.

- Epilepsy: This is a seizure disorder that stems from the brain. Thus, women with epilepsy are more likely to experience premature ovarian failure, which leads to early menopause. In the year 2001, a study was conducted among women with epilepsy, which revealed that about 41% of the participants in the study had premature menopause. Sources: Stephanie Watson et al 2019.

Sex and menopause

Most African Australian women don't understand that menopause transition impacts upon sex drive and desire, function and satisfaction.

It is important to understand that age plays a role in menopause transition, but the biological and psychological changes that occur in menopause are independently important, meaning that some changes are solely due to menopause, and are unrelated to increasing age. Sex drive in women who are in menopause, are influenced by physical and mental illness, medication a woman is undergoing, relationship quality, psycho-social stresses and environment where a woman lives.

Sex drive is an evolutionary imperative that varies from woman to woman; it is a highly complex area in women's health and far more complicated than for men. Sex drive and desire in biological males is more straight forward and sexual issues are largely mechanical and not psychological. In contrast, sexual drive and desire in females involves biological, physiological and psychological factors. It is believed that this is due to the different outcomes of sexual reproduction for men and women. In heterosexual sex, if successful in sexual reproductive terms, it may result in a nine-month pregnancy and years of parenthood.

Therefore, to meet evolutionary requirements to have a successful pregnancy and to increase offspring survival, the female sex drive and desire has a lot of safety checks involved, which include psychological factors such as a need for emotional connection and security, which are all driven by hormones.

In humans, some of us think that sex is only for procreation but it is also for pleasure, connection, and increased emotional intimacy; this implies that after the sexual reproductive stage of a woman's life, sex and sexual intimacy remain important. (Dr Nicola Gates, 2019, PP. 180-181)

This brings us to the question, "At what age does a woman stop being sexually active?" There is no one answer to this question. However, studies show that being sexually active depends on the individual woman. A research letter in JAMA Internal Medicine reports that women between the ages of 40 to 65 who place greater importance on sex are more likely to stay sexually active as they age.

Some women when they reach the stage of menopause, struggle emotionally; intimacy with people may be there but intimacy with her husband may have gone, and the thought of sex makes her skin crawl. The husband often notices this and may think the woman no longer loves him.

Sex drive and desire in menopause

Drive and desire are sensitive to any changes in females' reproductive hormones. In women, changes in sex drive and desire are always in response to menstrual cycle, oral contraception, pregnancy, post-partum state, breast-feeding and the menopausal transition.

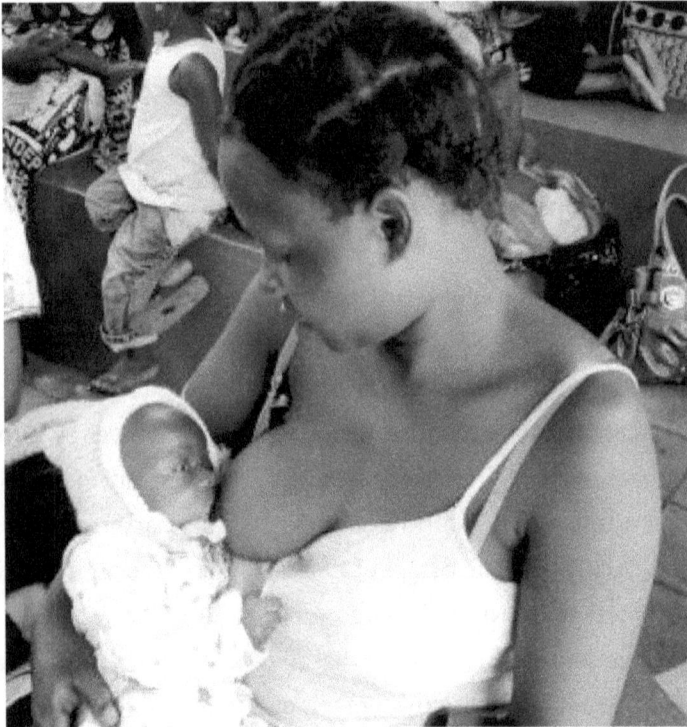

Figure: 33. Breastfeeding

Sex drive naturally declines with increasing age in both men and women. Biological sex drive as we know is all about reproduction and is very sensitive to age. As fertility goes down and the risk of birth defects and failed pregnancies increase, so the desire to procreate also goes down. When we were young, fit and healthy, our biological desire is to reproduce. But as we grow older, our biological material (genes) also grow older and our biological drive to procreate diminishes accordingly. The sex drive in women declines because of loss of androgens, including testosterone.

From conversations with men, I have heard that there are some men who have nine sexual intercourses a night and must have a very strong desire for sex. Contrary to this popular belief, experts say frequency of sexual intercourse has nothing to do with sexual desire or satisfaction. Kingsberg (2018) says that sexual desire is more than just an issue of low libido or sex drive, but it is rather the biological component of desire, which is reflected in spontaneous sexual interest including sexual thoughts, erotic fantasies, and daydreams.

As I mentioned before, we have sex for many reasons beside procreation and this includes fun, communication, tension release, affirmation, comfort, expression of love, to please a partner and to induce sleep. Oestrogen impacts on orgasms and tissues that are involved in sexual arousal, physiological responsiveness and satisfaction, including skin, breasts, muscles and urogenital organs. Loss of oestrogen therefore impacts on sexual function and satisfaction, as well as emotions associated with trust and security as well as stress.

"Scientifically, drive and desire both impact the female body's physiological responsiveness to sexual activity, sexual function and satisfaction. Sex drive is a hormonally determined biological function of the brain and in women is associated primarily with oestrogen androgens like testosterone. Sexual desire is a motivational state of interest in sexual activities and includes sex drive, feelings of trust and security, and pleasure." From Science

Other physical menopausal symptoms such as weight gain, fatigue, hot flushes and night sweats may also affect sexual desire in women. Nicola Gates (2019) observes that changes in sexual desire and function are compounded by unhelpful messages about sex and sexuality. We live in an increasingly sexualised society and as a result, the perception of what is normal is being skewed and there is increasing insecurity about sex drive and desire. More adults today think they may have a problematic loss of sexual drive and desire and are not having sexual intimacy at normal levels. There is no normal level of sexual intimacy and there is no standard or normal level of sex drive or desire. We all fall on a continuum from no drive to high drive and each of us move along the range or not, depending upon what we have mentioned above, that is hormones, age, life stage, individual, psychological, relationship and the environment we live in. (P. 185).

Here then comes a question, "If there is no standard or normal level of sex drive, what makes a problem?" In an attempt to answer this question, we can say that dissatisfaction of sex in a human being is entirely something subjective. So, if a person is not dissatisfied with sex life, there is no problem; it is only when a person is dissatisfied, is when a problem comes into existence. Similarly, sexual dysfunction is not a big problem unless it causes significant distress. The thought that sex might be nice, but one does not bother about it is not a big deal, we cannot call this as "sexual dysfunction", because this is common among women. A national investigation of Australian women in middle-age found that only thirty percent of women reported significant distress of sexual dysfunction because of their low sexual desire, which means they have sexual interest or arousal disorder. (Dr Nicola Gates, 2019). As I said before, I still want to emphasize that the important thing for us to consider in sex is that sexual desire naturally changes in both men and women, and not just with chronological age but in relationship and life stages too.

Sexual function in menopause

It appears African Australian women are uncertain about sexual function when they are in their menopause. Dr Nicola Gates (2019) notes that women, wherever they live, should know that beside sex drive and desire, menopause impacts on the sexual function of women. During puberty, women have oestrogen that increases vaginal lubrication and the plumpness of the vaginal walls. When oestrogen decreases during perimenopause and menopause, it impacts on the vagina and the whole urogenital environment. The immediate symptoms reported about urogenital deterioration are vaginal dryness, irritation and itching; they start with the onset of the menopause transition and are usually progressive in nature. The vaginal walls become drier, thinner and less elastic; the vulva, vagina and urinary tract will have a lower blood supply. These issues make sex painful and functionally difficult for women. Sex that hurts in an unwanted way is not conducive to desire and a national study in Australian, found that vaginal dryness and pain during or after sexual intercourse were significant factors contributing to low desire and sexual arousal disorder. Painful intercourse can also make a woman fearful of pain and increase anxiety, which can burden mental health, and further reduce desire for sex. Once a woman begins to avoid sex because of pain, this can lead to total loss of physical connection and finally to distress. (PP. 186-187).

▶ Studies found that pain during sex is common after menopause as oestrogen levels fall, which can cause the vagina to feel dry. This can affect a woman's desire for sex, but a woman can use osteoderm lubricants (See figure: 25)

Sexual satisfaction

Like sexual desire and function discussed above, sexual satisfaction in woman changes with menopause and age and also involves both physiological and emotional responses. Study shows that during the menopause transition, hormone changes decrease intensity of sexual orgasm that may reduce physiological satisfaction, but emotional intimacy needs may still be met. The bonding and social behaviour between a woman and a man is influenced by "oxytocin", commonly known as the "love hormone". The oxytocin works within the brain as well as influencing the woman's body. Oxytocin is usually thought of as a female hormone for lactation and levels do rise when women give birth. However, oxytocin also impacts multiple areas of the reproductive system and behaviour such as bonding, sex drive and orgasm. During the menopausal transition, and afterwards, the lowered levels of oestrogen reduce oxytocin production in the brain, and this can lower sexual satisfaction or relationship satisfaction including feelings of security. (Nicola Gates, 2019, P. 189).

If penetrative sex becomes painful, and stops being satisfying, look for alternatives as to how you could have sex. Thus, with menopause and age, new considerations for sexual pleasure could be clitoral stimulation or oral sex, instead of vaginal penetration sex. And if there are differences in orgasms (libido), the best option for a woman to use is masturbation to maintain satisfaction without overburdening the relationship. (Nicola gates, 2019).

"The pelvic floor includes muscles, ligaments and connective tissues that support the pelvic organs such as bladder, uterus, vagina and rectum. When a woman's pelvic floor muscles contract during sex, she lifts those organs and the vagina, anus and urethra sphincters tighten, which closes their opening and stops urine or wind escaping. The pelvic floor is crucial for sexual function. However, pregnancies and childbirth, and surgeries weaken the pelvic floor. Menopausal changes also affect the pelvic floor." Source: from Science

Conversations about sex and sexual satisfaction between couples require a healthy positive relationship to support honest, respectful communication, and such conversations will further build the depth and intimacy of the relationship. Changes in sex and intimacy can be very challenging and confronting for some couples as they may discover that there is not enough emotional glue of kindness, respect, support and healthy communication between them.

Oestrogen, the brain and cognition

Oestrogen is an essential brain player, maintaining brain health and function throughout the entire lifespan. Nicola Gates (2019) pointed out that oestrogen has a direct role in prenatal development growth in puberty and hormonal changes throughout adulthood, including menopause and old age. It is used throughout the brain by brain cells called neurons, the support cells in the brain called astrocytes, and to maintain brain-tissue-specific function.

"The finding of research indicates that the action of oestrogen in the brain is controlled by two receptor systems (1) Sexual reproduction and behaviour (2) Brain function." From Science bite

Oestrogen helps protect brain functions, such as reducing free radicals and influencing genes that control how neurons adapt, generate and grow. Thus, when we learn new things, such as a new language or how to operate a new machine, our brain makes changes. Keeping our brain stimulated and challenged, leads to brain growth and builds brain reserve, which makes the brain resilient. In this way, oestrogen helps protect the brain by helping it to be neuroplastic. (P. 127).

Menopause, memory and dementia

As we have discussed before, oestrogen influences memory and the brain structures associated with memory. Nicola Gates (2019) notes, that low levels of oestrogen mean low levels of specific neurotransmitters required for memory formation, which reduces the amount of information transfer and consolidation. Since oestrogen impacts memory, the links to cognitive decline and dementia are unavoidable. Dementia is certainly a terrifying prospect, but having a cognitive change during menopause is not the same as having dementia. The cognitive changes associated with menopause are most likely just part of the transition, which is temporary, deterioration rarely continues a downward trajectory, and the difficulties are not usually so severe as to constitute an impairment. Menopause memory changes are temporary and not severe. The different between menopause and dementia comes down to cause. (PP. 132-133)

"Oestrogen decline leads to lower levels of enzymes necessary for memory.

Choline acetyltransferase is an enzyme required for the synthesis of acetylcholine; a neurotransmitter associated with memory function. Specifically, with lower levels of acetylcholine the nerve cells in the hippocampal memory structure have fewer spines for communication, which means less information transfer in memory. Oestrogen, therefore, has a neuroprotective role and we want to know how the introduction of exogenous oestrogen may improve memory and reduce dementia risk." From: Science

When women enter menopause, they are getting older. The brain naturally undergoes age-related changes, so it can be tricky to isolate which changes are caused by age and which may be due to menopausal hormonal changes. However, some functions such as their general knowledge and vocabulary in fact continue to steadily increase as the woman gets older. Dementia is not normal brain ageing but is due to a disease process. Dementia is an umbrella term which includes many different types of neurological diseases, it is now called a "neurocognitive disorder" and there are various types of dementia which I cannot mention them all here due to shortness of space in this book.

Intimate Relationships

Studies show that men's and women's needs of intimate relationships change over time as they go through reproductive life and lifespan. The studies revealed that although menopause is an important milestone in women's development, it may have less impact on women's general health and happiness than their intimate relationships.

It is confirmed by psychologists that good-quality relationships are crucial to women's wellbeing, and many of them value intimate relationships in their entire life. Relationship quality can either contribute to or diminish a woman's capacity to cope with all aspects of life including health challenges and menopause. The best example found in research is that a supportive relationship reduces the negative impact of breast cancer and increases adjustment and coping.

When we talk about "relationship quality" we mean to say what attract a partner, such as trust, security, good communication, respect, conflict resolution, sexual expression as well as the right age for a relationship. These factors have more impact on desire than on menopause.

The difference between the women who are and who are not concerned about the changes in their sex live, is largely due to their relationship status quality, as well as their difference that attributes towards sex and relationships. We have discussed before that menopausal sexual satisfaction is directly related to relationship satisfaction, and not to menopause as many might think. In these studies, sexual satisfaction was not defined as "sexual intercourse" but rather as "satisfaction" with how sexuality was expressed within the relationship. Most women think that changes in their sex life are not a significant issue at all. For example, not many women are concerned with a change in their libido due to menopause.

Level of support impacts on relationship quality and feeling unsupported is a factor that significantly inhibits desire. Research suggests that an increase in the quality of emotional intimacy within the relationship and increased domestic support from one's partner increases sexual desire. (Dr Nicola Gates, 2019).

As the couple go through their relationship, the biological drive for sex or procreation diminishes and some relationships here can become stuck if there is insufficient or inadequate desire.

Dr Nicola Gates (2019) observes that in one study, where over two hundred women were questioned regarding their marriage, stress and menopause, the response from the women revealed that an unsatisfying marriage left women more vulnerable to stress and they had more menopause symptoms, than those women in satisfying relationships. Those women in unsatisfying marriages were found with symptoms of sleep disturbance and hot flushes due to an unsatisfactory relationship.

With increasing age and menopause, the relationship focusses shifts to a more related connection and transformational enrichment. Studies suggest that this increases desire for companionship and intimacy and requires reconsideration for support for future dreams and shared interests.

Becoming and remaining well-partnered, takes time and effort but bestows multiple benefits. Unfortunately, the contrary is also true. People in unhealthy, unhappy or unsatisfying relationships have reduced health, lower quality of life and shorter lifespans. Being unhappy in a relationship is more detrimental than being single, divorced or widowed.

Chapter Nine
Not Getting Pregnant

Why am I not getting pregnant?

Some of the African Australian women, beside looking for money and sexual pleasure, also search for a new baby or babies, which is aimed to boost their financial conditions through the Family Tax Benefit Part A and B in Centrelink. During a year or two of sugar relationships, some women try hard to get pregnant; some of them do have children but with others nothing happens. This makes a woman who does not get pregnant, sometimes to ask herself, "Why am I not getting pregnant?" There are many reasons why a woman may not get pregnant after a long time of trying. Study shows that some couples may conceive the very first month they try, and approximately 75% will get pregnant within six months of the relationship. How long it may take for a woman to get pregnant depends on how frequently she is having sex; if a woman is having sex during her most fertile days or during her early womanhood, she is most likely to get pregnant.

Between 10 and 15 percent of couples will experience infertility. This means they will not conceive after one year of trying. Of these infertile couples, approximately one-third will discover fertility problems are on the woman's side, another third will find the problem is on the man's side, and the rest will find problems on both sides.

Rachel Gurevich (2019) observes that sometimes irregularities and structural problems in the reproduction system may be due to a low sperm count or underlying medical problems. However, the truth is that most infertility issues in women are silent, while male infertilities have rare symptoms. Therefore, Rachel Gurevich came to the conclusion that there are eight possible reasons why a woman may not get pregnant after months or years of trying. The eight reasons include the following: -

I. The man may be sleeping too much:

► One of the reasons a woman may not get pregnant is that they don't have frequent sexual intercourse because the man is sleeping too much and the woman does not want to interrupt his sleep. However, it is important to know that many couples won't conceive right away. Scientists report that about 80 percent of couples who have frequent sex, get pregnant after six months of trying and approximately 90 percent of women get pregnant after 12 months. This assumes that the couples have "well-timed intercourse" every month.

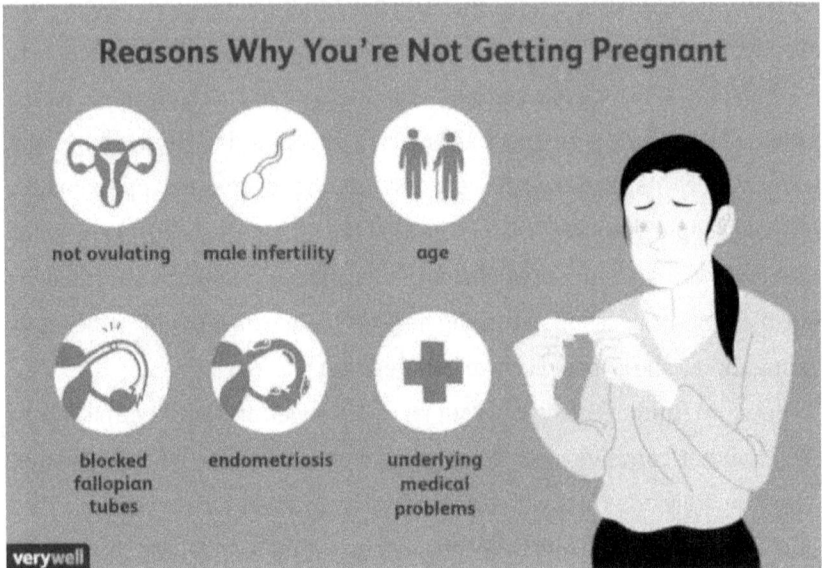

Source: Rachel Gurevich (2019)

II. Not ovulating:

▸ In human beings, for a conception to occur it requires an egg and sperm. Therefore, if a woman is not ovulating, there will never be a pregnancy. Some African men and women keep on blaming each other for not being productive, without understanding that things such as being over or under weight or having primary ovarian insufficiency may attribute to the no conception. According to scientists, most women who are experiencing ovulation problems have irregular periods. However, regular menstrual cycles don't guarantee that ovulation is occurring. Ovulation is a common cause of female infertility and it can be triggered by many conditions. Polycystic ovarian symptoms (PCOS) is one of the most common causes of female infertility, affecting an estimated five million women around the globe (approximately 8% of total world population of women). Polycystic ovary syndrome is a hormonal disorder causing enlarged ovaries with small cysts on the outer edges of ovary, but doctors don't know exactly what causes PCOS.

▸ Women with PCOS often have polycystic ovaries. This means that the ovaries have many tiny, benign and painless cysts. Nevertheless, a woman can get pregnant with PCOS. Most women can conceive by a combination of lifestyle changes and fertility drugs. However, women with PCOS do have an increased risk for pregnancy complications. They are more likely to develop gestational diabetes, pregnancy related to high blood pressure and pre-term labour. Babies born to women with PCOS have an increased risk of needing NICU care after birth.

▸ It is reported that some women with PCOS struggle with obesity. Studies have found that losing some of the extra weight may bring back ovulation. According to the research, losing 5 to 10 percent of a woman's current weight may be enough to jump-start her menstrual cycles. Losing weight is not easy for anybody, and it may be even more difficult for those with PCOS. The study also found that women with PCOS usually have high levels of androgen hormones in their bodies;

scientifically androgens are found both in men and women, although androgens are considered male hormones. Therefore, one of the main reasons why the women with PCOS can't conceive is because they don't ovulate, or they don't ovulate regularly.

Dr Len Kliman (2020) observes that polycystic ovarian syndrome or PCOS is a prevalent, hormone-based condition. It is an illness that affects numerous women across the world. People with polycystic ovarian syndrome have an imbalance in their hormone production. The out-of-whack hormones affect the body in multiple different ways and cause numerous symptoms to manifest, signalling the onset of PCOS. From the nature and frequency of the menstrual cycle to body-hair growth patterns and skin quality, this condition produces mild discomfort in the best-case scenario and may get moderately incapacitating in severe cases.

The followings are *symptoms of polycystic ovarian syndrome:-*

- ▸ Infertility
- ▸ Irregular or absent ovulation
- ▸ Amenorrhea (absence of monthly menstrual cycles) or oligomenorrhea (irregular monthly menstrual cycles)
- ▸ Recurrent miscarriage
- ▸ Abnormal hair growth, also known as hirsutism, found on the upper lip, chin, around the nipples, or on the abdomen.
- ▸ Acne
- ▸ Especially oily skin and hair
- ▸ Male pattern balding
- ▸ Obesity
- ▸ The presence of polycystic ovaries during ultrasound examination
- ▸ Insulin resistance
- ▸ High levels of androgens, also known as hyperandrogenism
- ▸ And elevated level of the hormones LH.

I have heard a lot during my lifetime that some women may have a child, but then they find it hard to get pregnant a second time. Many of us don't know that secondary infertility is the inability to conceive or carry a pregnancy following the delivery of a child. This is something not uncommon among women, and according to Dr Austin (2017) a woman who already has had a child, is likely to have a successful second pregnancy. But some women although they have already had a child, during sugar relationships or even during their second remarriage, they do not get pregnant. Unfortunately such women hardly ever admit that they are infertile. As a result, they keep on telling lies to their men that they were pregnant and they have had a miscarriage, purely to keep their relationships. Furthermore, other women tell lies to their men that they were pregnant, and then went to the doctors to help them remove the child, because they are not prepared to go ahead with the pregnancy.

III. The problem is with him, not me (Male infertility)

Experience shows that most women usually can carry a baby, but it takes time before coming pregnant. It is reported that of between 20-30 percent of infertile couples, fertility factors are on the man's side, and 40 percent of infertility factors are found on both sides.

According to the American Society of Reproductive Medicine, one-third of infertility cases in couples are due to female infertility, and another one-third is due to male infertility and the remaining third is due to both sides.

IV. Age-related infertility is causing a problem:

▶ It is generally believed that getting pregnant after the age of 35 is more difficult than for the age 25, but it is not impossible. According to the Centre for Disease Control and Prevention, it is found that 30 percent of women aged 40-44 will experience infertility. Therefore, only 5 percent of women, who pass 40, have a chance of getting pregnant.

▶ Male fertility does change with age; a man may have the impression that age only matters with female fertility. While the change in fertility is more drastic in women, men have biological clocks, too.

- One research study was conducted at Soroka University in Israel about semen quality in normal males, and research compared the quantity and quality of semen to the men's ages. At the end of the day, researchers found that semen quantity peaked between the men's ages of 30 — 35. On the other end of the spectrum, overall semen quantity was found to be lowest after age 55. This study also found that sperm motility changed with age. Sperm motility is how well the sperm can swim. It is believed that sperm motility is best before age 25 and lowest after age 55.

- Some women assume that because they are still getting regular periods their fertility is fine, but this is not true. Age impacts egg quality as well as quantity in women, as we have discussed before.

- If the husband is five or more years older than the wife/partner, this can increase the woman's risk of fertility problems after the age of 35. However, the African experiences prove that the study could be wrong on this point, because in African communities, especially in South Sudan, the age variance of some married couples can be huge. For example, a man aged 40 could marry a woman aged 18 or 25 and a man aged 60 years could marry a woman aged 20 or 30, yet they produce many children. Therefore, from my research, this area of age-related infertility needs further study.

- Fallopian tubes may be blocked:

- Studies discovered that 25-30 percent of female infertility cases are caused by irregular ovulation. The rest of female infertility cases are caused by blocked fallopian tubes, uterine structural problems, or endometriosis.

- For the sake of those who may not know, the fallopian tubes are the pathway between women's ovaries and the uterus. The fallopian tubes are not directly attached to ovaries. Sperm must swim up from the cervix (see figure 22), through the uterus, and into the fallopian tubes. The cervix is a small rubber ball about 3 centimetres or one inch in diameter; and the uterus is made up of three layers: the serosa, the myometrium, and the endometrium. The serosa is the outer skin of the uterus, it secretes a watery fluid to prevent friction between the uterus and nearby organs; the myometrium is the middle uterine layer, it is the thickest layer of uterus; and the myometrium is made up of thick smooth muscle tissue.

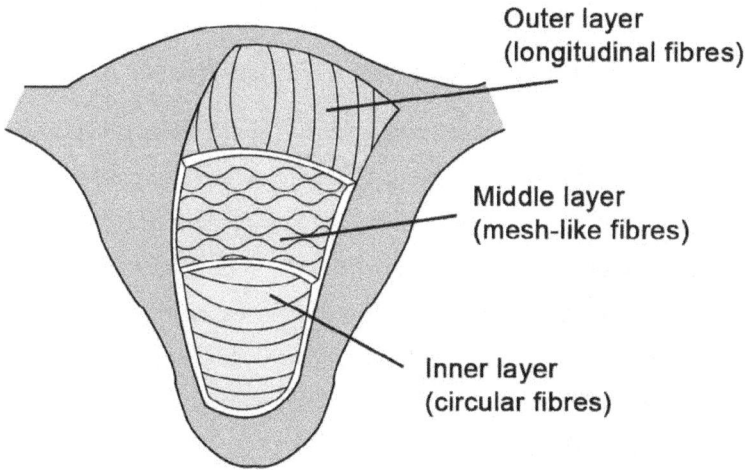

Outer layer
(longitudinal fibres)

Middle layer
(mesh-like fibres)

Inner layer
(circular fibres)

Figure: 34. Showing three layers of uterus

▸ When an egg is released from the ovaries, hair-like projections from the fallopian tube draw the egg into fallopian tube, where the sperm and egg meet. When an obstruction prevents the egg from travelling down the tube, a woman can be said to have a blocked fallopian tube, also known as tubal factor infertility. This can occur on one side or both sides of fallopian tubes and is the cause of infertility in up to 30 percent of infertile women.

▸ However, if something prevents the fallopian tubes from functioning properly, or if anything blocks the sperm or egg from meeting, the woman won't be able to get pregnant. It is said that there are many possible causes of blocked fallopian tubes. The most common cause is pelvic inflammatory disease (PID) which is an infection of reproductive organs, occurring when bacteria travels through the cervix to the uterus and fallopian tube. PID can cause infertility, ectopic pregnancy, chronic pelvic pain, tubal or ovarian abscesses, adhesions, peritonitis and peri-hepatitis. Pelvic inflammation can be acute (sudden or severe symptoms), chronic or silent (no symptoms). It has been discovered that PID is usually caused by sexual transmitted disease (STDs). The common causes include chlamydia and gonorrhoea.

V: The woman has endometriosis

A woman may not get pregnant because she has endometriosis, 1 in 10 women suffer from endometriosis, with 1 in 3 likely to present with infertility. The endometriosis is the inner lining of the uterus. In other words, we can say endometriosis is a condition resulting from the appearance of endometrial tissue outside the uterus and causing pelvic pain, especially associated with menstruation. Each month, the endometrium thickens and renews itself, preparing for pregnancy. If pregnancy does not occur, the endometrium sheds in a process known as "menstruation".

Conditions that involve the endometrium and that may impact women's fertility include the following: -

- ▶ Too thin or too thick endometrium
- ▶ Luteal phase defect, which is the portion of a woman's menstrual cycle that occurs after ovulation but before the first day of her next menstrual cycle. On average, the luteal phase lasts between 10 -14 days.
- ▶ Endometriosis, this is endometrium-like tissue that grows in places outside of the uterus. It is an abnormal and often painful disorder that affects anywhere from six percent to ten percent of women. The overgrowth of tissue is only part of the reason why endometriosis interferes with fertility.
- ▶ Adenomyosis
- ▶ Asherman's syndrome (which means uterine adhesions). Adhesions are abnormal bands of scar tissue that join organs or parts of organs that

are not normally joined. Adhesions may cause infertility by preventing the egg and sperm from meeting, interfering with ovulation and making the uterus inhospitable to a fertilised embryo. Adhesions are one possible cause of blocked fallopian tubes.

- ▶ Viral infection
- ▶ Endometrial cancer is sometimes known as uterine cancer. The most common symptoms of endometrial cancer are unusual vaginal bleeding, either in between periods or after a woman has been through menopause. An abnormal watery discharge or bloody pain during sexual intercourse are common symptoms of endometrial cancer.
- ▶ It is estimated that up to 50 percent of women with endometriosis will have difficulty getting pregnant. It is also reported that in the later stages of the disease, a woman may experience pelvic pain, weight loss, and an ability to feel a mass in her pelvis. In other words, most common symptoms of endometriosis are having painful periods and pelvic pain at times besides menstruation (as we have just discussed above). However, not all women with endometriosis have these symptoms; some women have discovered they have endometriosis as part of infertility in their lives.

VI. There is an underlying medical problem

From medical research, it is revealed that underlying conditions can also lead to

- ▶ infertility in both men and women. For example, a thyroid imbalance or undiagnosed
- ▶ diabetes can lead to infertility. Infertility and depression often go together. So one should not be surprised that infertility can lead to depression; therefore, women who experience depression is more likely to have fertility problems. Similarly, women who have struggled trying to conceive, may have depression during pregnancy, as well as depression after pregnancy (known as postpartum depression).

In this contemporary world, our lives depend on medications. However, some people stop taking their medications because they think it is not right for them. Here is strong message for all of us, "Never stop taking a medication without talking to your doctor first." When talking to your doctor, let him/her know that you are trying to get pregnant.

Interestingly, one of my informants, a female aged 46, says, "I have one grown-up child and I have been trying to get pregnant in the last twenty years. I have seen medical doctors together with my husband, and the doctor said that the problem is with my husband. After seeing the doctor, I have tried to get pregnant with other men outside marriage, but nothing happened. So I am wondering why I am not getting pregnant?" I told her, "I am not a medical person, but from my reading and from your narratives, it seems you have *polycystic ovary syndrome* because it has been reported that a woman who has *polycystic ovary syndrome* may not have second child.

Polycystic ovary syndrome is a hormonal imbalance that can disrupt ovulation and is usually a common cause of secondary (or primary) infertility.

We have discussed before that if a woman does not ovulate, she won't be able to get pregnant. Most women who are experiencing ovulation problems have irregular periods.

VII. Unexplained infertility:

Studies found that between 25 to 30 percent of infertile couples never find out why the wife can't get pregnant. Unexplained infertility is a frustrating diagnosis of undiscovered problems. This is a common problem with women. It is said, one in four fertility-challenged couples may be told that there is no explanation for why they can't conceive. This does not mean they have no options — but all of these depend on their ages.

Orgasmic disorders in men and women

A number of disorders in males and females are associated with orgasm; this can lead to distress, frustration, and feelings of shame, for both of them.

Erectile dysfunction in males

Before we go deep into examining erectile dysfunction in males, we need to know what is meant by the term "Erectile Dysfunction" and then we should understand that erectile dysfunction is more common than we think. The erectile dysfunction (ED) can be defined as "The inability to attain or maintain an erection of the penis in males" to produce adequate sexual satisfaction for both partners. In other words, ED could be defined as the inability to get or keep an erection for satisfactory sexual performance. The erectile dysfunction typically worsens over time and can progress from mild to complete impotence, if not treated appropriately. If you are concerned about erectile dysfunction, you must know that you are not alone.

It is estimated 1 in 10 men has a problem related to having sex, such as premature ejaculation or erectile dysfunction. Sexual problems can affect any man, whether he is straight, gay, bisexual or transgender. A man may think that he is the only one in the world who experiences erectile dysfunction but this is not true. Most men experience it at some time in their life, and Urologists have discovered that erectile dysfunction is caused by physical or psychological factors mainly in men over 50 years.

Erectile dysfunction is most common among men over 50 years of age, and this is caused by several factors. One of the factors is "an aging man's lifestyle and behaviour" and "androgen deficiency", these often decrease testosterone levels in men, and affect sexual function. David F. Mobley (2016) states a study was conducted between men age 30-79 years, which revealed that 24 percent of the men who underwent the study, were found to have had testosterone levels below 300ng/dl and 5.6 percent of them had symptomatic androgen deficiency. The same study also found that men age 57-64 years have their sexual activities decreased by 73 percent, while men aged 75-85 years have their sexual activities increased by 26 percent. For some men, this represents a problem, but for others it does not.

Changes and loss of function in organs within the human body is normal and is a consequence of the ageing process. This is also true with the endocrine system, when the level of testosterone production in the testicles goes down. The decrease in testosterone means a decrease in erections of the penis making erection not as frequent and rigid as compared to a young man's erectile function. Although these changes are in themselves not life threatening, they can impact on their libido and desire to engage in sexual activity. Study also found that most female partners undergo menopause at 52 years of age with a significant decline in a man's relations as a partner.

Urologists have discovered that erectile dysfunctions are caused by physical factors in men over 50 years. However, it appears that most erectile dysfunction in older men is caused by a blockage of blood-flow to the penis, commonly caused by atherosclerosis and diabetes. Some medical doctors discovered that erectile dysfunction can also be caused by a faulty vein, which lets blood drain too quickly from the penis while other physicians discovered that it is caused by physical disorders and hormonal imbalances. Hormonal imbalances occur when there is too much or too little of a hormone in the bloodstream.

Most older men from age 50, suffer not from ED but from erection dissatisfaction. It is reported that men aged 50 who smoke or have diabetes, have erection changes. This change is gradual in some men but in others, it happens more quickly. Dr Newton says ED does not follow many of the medical condition trends. According to him, the followings are some of the main causes of ED: -

- ▸ Low testosterone: A man with low testosterone may notice symptoms such as fatigue, depression, decreased interest in sexual intercourse, changes in muscle mass and changes in body hair on his body.
- ▸ Diabetes: Diabetes is one of the most frequent causes of erectile dysfunction as the body can't appropriately handle sugar.
- ▸ Peripheral vascular disease: This is when a man has peripheral vascular disease, which leads to the narrowing of blood vessels and subsequently causes erectile dysfunction.
- ▸ Obesity: A man who is too fat often experiences erectile dysfunction.
- ▸ Psycho-social stress: This is when a man is too concerned about erectile

dysfunction, which often leads to mild erectile dysfunction and in a long term could lead to constant erectile dysfunction.

▸ Smoking: Medically it is found that stopping smoking can help reduce the risk of multiple medical conditions, including erectile dysfunction.

It is said when a man becomes sexually aroused, hormones, muscles, nerves, and blood vessels all work with one another to create an erection. At this time, nerve signals are sent from the brain to the penis, to stimulate muscles or to relax. This in turn, allows blood to flow to the tissue in the penis. According to a 2005 Journal of Sexual Medicine, a study was conducted among 500 couples across Europe and USA, and it was discovered that the average erection during sex lasts 5.4 minutes. But normal erections can last anywhere from 30 minutes to one hour or even longer. The study also discovered that the flow of blood in the penis causes either a weak or strong erection. Scientists found that weak erections are normally caused by the hardening of arteries, high blood pressure, high cholesterol or diabetes.

In younger men, psychological problems are the likeliest reason for erectile dysfunction. It appears the sexual difficulties in young men may be linked to depression, fatigue, stress, feelings of inadequacy, personal sexual fears, rejection by parents or friends or peers and finally erectile dysfunction in young men can be caused by the memory of sexual abuse in childhood.

It is generally believed that ageing does not affect sexual activity in men, but is likely to affect women. Study found that a man 55 years old can expect to be sexually active for another7 years. This means that men can be sexually active up to age 62 years. However, other scholars found that a man of 55 years can be sexually active for another 15 years, which means men can be sexually active up to 70 years old. On the other side of the coin, study found that a woman aged 55 years can be sexually active for another 11 years. Which means women can be sexually active up to the age of 66 years old.

Generally, it is believed that an increase in age for both men and women leads to a decrease in sexual activity. It is reported that 46 percent of men aged 65-70 years are sexually active, as compared to 39 percent of men aged

71-75 years; the same comparison was made for men aged 76-80 years and it was found that only 25 percent of them were sexually active. Study also found that 51 percent of mature men are sexually active as compare to 31 percent of mature women.

In a separate development, the researchers in Europe and America surveyed a group of women between 40 to 100 years old, with a medium age of 67. Research discovered that half of the responders said they were sexually active, and most of the women said they were able to become aroused, maintaining lubrication and achieve orgasm during sex, even after the age of 80 years. However, the same study found that about half of men aged 40 to 70 have erectile dysfunction (ED) to some degree, although only one in ten reported a complete inability to have erections. With modern medicines, taking drugs for erectile dysfunction can help 70 percent of healthy men. Nearly every primary care physician internist and geriatrician today understands that many older men remain interested in sexual activity as they age.

Sildenafil (Viagra) is often the first drug that doctors usually prescribe to their patients when they are experiencing sexual dysfunction. The second drug your doctor may prescribe is Tadalafil (Cialis). These drugs have been on the market for a long time and their side effects and other medications and food that interact with them are well known. The only obstacle that patients could find is that the cost of Viagra tablets is somewhat expensive, and the cost of Cialis is too expensive for low income earners. You must visit your doctor to get this drug as it can't be bought over the counter.

Vardenafil (Viagra) is effective for 12 hours, while Tadalafil (Cialis) is effective for 36 hours. Both drugs you can take with or without food at least one or two hours before sexual intercourse. A newer form of the drug that dissolves on the tongue might work faster than the pill a man can swallow.

The treatment of ED is not something new, it started in the time of the Yellow Emperor's rule which ended around 200 B.C. At that time men were using traditional Chinese medicine. Nearly one thousand years later, the Egyptians Papyrus Ebers, which was documented around 1600 B.C. cured impotence with a mixture of crocodile hearts and wood oil that was applied on the penis.

The modern medicine for the treatment of impotence was invented in 1973 and this medicine is still used up until today by urologists. The breakthrough occurred in 1998 when Sildenafil (Viagra) became the first oral drug to be approved to treat ED. This was followed by the usage of Tadalafil (Cialis) in 2003 (David F. Mobley, 2016). The introduction of anti-impotence treatment in the last few years has spurred more research into the cause of sexual dysfunction among both men and women, and effective therapies are now available to help put the lust back into men's and women's lives.

Today, medical doctors help men who have erectile dysfunctions by first prescribing Viagra 5 mg, and if it does not work, the doctor changes to Cialis 5 mg. But what is Viagra and Cialis? We can define both Viagra and Cialis as medication used to treat erectile dysfunction (impotence) and symptoms of benign prostatic hypertrophy (enlarged prostate) in men. It is taken by mouth or injection into a vein.

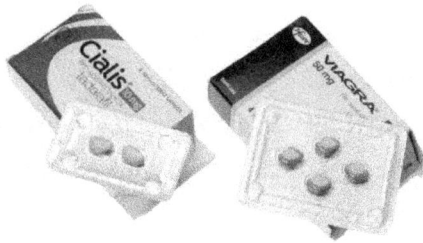

Figure: 35. Male Cialis and Viagra

It is recommended that a man takes one tablet of either Viagra or Cialis daily; it must be taken at approximately the same time every day, without regard to the timing of sexual activity. However, the difference between the two drugs is on how long each of them stay in the system. Cialis provides penile hardness for over a longer period than Viagra. Medically, it is reported that both Cialis and Viagra take about 30-60 minutes to start working in a man's blood system. Researchers recommend that a man should take Viagra or Cialis at least 1-2 hours before he plans to have sex. The effects of Cialis may last up to 36 hours, while Viagra only last 12 hours.

It has been observed by many health professionals that Cialis and Viagra increase testosterone levels and Cialis increases blood flow to the penis enabling an erection to occur when a man is sexually stimulated.

It is believed that men with low testosterone levels do not live as long as men with normal testosterone levels.

The maximum recommended dose of Cialis is one 20 mg tablet taken before sexual activity. A man with kidney disease should take only 10 mg Cialis tablet and later may be increased to 20 mg. The recommended dose for Cialis for ED is 10 mg, taken at least 30 minutes before sexual activity. Dosage may be increased to 20 mg or decreased to 5 mg based on efficacy and tolerability.

Drinking small amounts of wine or beer is unlikely to affect Cialis or cause any health risks. But excessive drink, while taking Cialis, can lead to orthostatic hypotension. (Orthostatic hypotension is a form of low blood pressure that happens when you stand up from sitting or lying down, and can make a person feel dizzy or lightheaded, and even faint).

Therefore, it is advisable that any man taking Cialis when he goes to a doctor, should tell the doctor that he is currently taking Cialis to avoid the doctor from prescribing nitrate medications that would make the man feel dizzy, faint, have a heart attack or stroke.

Female sexual dysfunction

What is female sexual dysfunction?

We can define female sexual dysfunction as a problem that occurs when a woman is being prevented from sexually responding to having a satisfying orgasm. From the medical point of view, persistent, recurrent problems with sexual response, desire, orgasm or pain that distress a woman with a partner is known as sexual dysfunction. Many women experience problems with sexual dysfunction at some point, and some have difficulties throughout their lives.

Female sexual dysfunction can occur at any stage of life of a woman. It can occur only in certain or in all sexual situations. Female sexual dysfunction is complex and is a poorly understood condition that affects women of all ages. Female sexual complaints are common, occurring in approximately 40 percent of women. Most of these women complain of decreased desired in sex.

According to researchers, over 66 percent of women have had some type of sexual dysfunction. The most common problem reported was hypoactive sexual desire disorder (HSDD) or lack of sexual desire. Loss of sexual desire, known in medical terms as HSDD, is the most common form of sexual dysfunction among women of all ages. A recent study showed that nearly one-third of women aged 18 to 59 suffer from a loss of interest in sex. Another study revealed that about 25 percent of women aged between 21 and 30 of age experience hypoactive sexual disorder. In the same report, it was found that approximately 89 percent of women over 80 years old were also experiencing hypoactive sexual disorder. All-in-all the above findings inform us that sexual dysfunction is common among women of all ages.

Unlike men's main sexual complaint, which is erectile dysfunction, women's biggest sexual problem is caused by a combination of both mental and physical factors as we shall discuss after under "painful intercourse".

What are the symptoms of female sexual dysfunction?

Sexual dysfunction symptoms in women vary from one person to the other depending on what type of sexual dysfunction one is experiencing. The common symptoms of female sexual dysfunction include:-

- ► Low sexual desire: This symptom is common in women and it involves a lack of interest and willingness to have sex
- ► Sexual arousal disorder: A woman may have a desire for sex, but she finds it difficult to be aroused or to maintain arousal during sexual intercourse.

- Orgasmic disorder: This is when a woman finds it difficult to achieve orgasm after sufficient sexual arousal and ongoing stimulation.
- Sexual pain disorders: This is when a woman has pain associated with sexual stimulation or vaginal contact.

What causes female sexual dysfunction?

It is worth mentioning that both men and women are affected by sexual dysfunction, as we have seen in males above. Sexual dysfunction occurs in adults of all ages, but those who are commonly affected are older adults; and this may be related to a decline in health associated with ageing.

It appears that many women are experiencing female sexual hypoactive, but they do not know what causes these problems in them. Studies found that sexual dysfunction in women could be caused by many factors, and the most common causes include:

- Inhibited Sexual Desire: Inhibited sexual desire is when a woman lacks sexual desire and has lost interest in sex. Sexual dysfunction in women can be a result of physical, psychological or social problems. We cannot overemphasise that a woman who is affected with lack of sexual desire may not want to involve in conversations about sex, because she takes this as exposing her weakness to others. Boredom with regular sexual routines may also contribute to a lack of enthusiasm for sex, as can lifestyle factors such as being in a career or being a childcare worker. In conventional usage, boredom is an emotional and occasionally psycho-logical state experienced when an individual is left without anything in particular to do, is not interested in their surroundings, or may feel that a day or period is dull, tedious or boring.
- Physical Causes: Studies found that there are many factors that contrib-ute to the physical cause of sexual dysfunction in women. These condi-tions include hormonal imbalance. (Hormones play an important role in regulating sexual function in women. With the decrease in the female hormone oestrogen that is related to ageing and menopause, many

women experience some changes in sexual function as they age, including poor vaginal lubrication and decreased genital sensation.) Hormone levels change after giving birth and during breastfeeding, kidney disease, liver failure, alcoholism or drug abuse, pregnancy, disorders of the genitalia and urinary system such as cystitis, and low oestrogen levels after menopause may lead to changes in sexual responsiveness. In addition, the side effects of certain medications such as antidepressant drugs, can affect sexual desire and function in some women. Blood pressure and chemotherapy (which is used in the treatment of cancer) can also affect sexual desire.

► Psychological and Social Causes: Female sexual dysfunction can also be caused through psychological and social factors, which are related to stress, anxiety, fatigue, when a woman is concerned about sexual performance, when a woman has marital or relationship problems with her husband or sugar daddy, fear of intimacy due to experience of abuse, depression, feelings of guilt or when a woman has been affected with past sexual trauma, cultural influence and poor body image of the man who wants to have sex with her.

► Inability to become aroused: Many people say that inability for a woman to become physically aroused during sexual intercourse is often due to insufficient vaginal lubrication. This inability may also be related to anxiety or to adequate stimulation as we have just discussed previously, under sub-title "psychological and social causes". In addition, contemporary researchers are investigating on how blood flow problems are affecting the vagina and clitoris not to be aroused.

► Lack of Orgasm (anorgasmia): This is the absence of sexual climax (orgasm). It is usually caused by a woman's sexual inhibition because of being inexperienced and lacking knowledge of how to have sex; lack of orgasm in a woman can also be caused by certain psychological factors such as feelings of guilt, anxiety, or recalling a past sexual trauma or abuse as we have discussed under sub-title "psychological and social causes" of female sexual dysfunction. Other factors contributing to anorgasmia include insufficient stimulation, effects of certain medications that a woman may be taking and chronic diseases in the body.

► Painful intercourse: Pain during intercourse can be caused by several problems, including endometriosis, a pelvic mass, ovarian cysts, vaginitis, poor lubrication of the vagina, the presence of scar tissue from surgery, or a sexual transmitted disease.

► A condition called vaginismus is a painful, involuntary spasm of the muscles that surround the vaginal entrance. (We can say a woman has vaginismus, when her vagina's muscles squeeze or spasm when the penis is entering it. Painful sex is often a woman's first sign that she has vaginismus.) It may occur in women who fear that penetration of the penis in their bodies will be painful and this often stems from a sexual phobia or from a previous traumatic or painful experience. In short, we can say that vaginismus is a condition which can be caused by physical stresses, emotional stresses, or both. It can become anticipatory, so that it happens because the person expects it to happen. Emotional triggers of vaginismus are many which include fear of pain or fear of pregnancy, anxiety of becoming guilty, an abusive relationship with a partner, recalling traumatic life events e.g. rape and sexual abuse.

► Physical triggers of Vaginismus are also many and these include infection e.g. urinary tract infection, poor health condition when a woman has cancer, former childbirth, menopause, when a woman has had pelvic surgery, when a man penetrates a woman's vagina before having adequate foreplay, when a woman has insufficient vagina lubrication, when a woman is taking certain medication that could cause her pain during sexual intercourse.

Can female sexual dysfunction be cured?

In the old days there was no cure for female sexual dysfunction, but today it can be cured. Although there are many types of medication, the majority of medical doctors seem to approve of Addyi® as the best medication to be used for the treatment of hypoactive sexual desire disorder (HSDD). They have recommended that only women who are premenopausal are candidates for using Addy®.

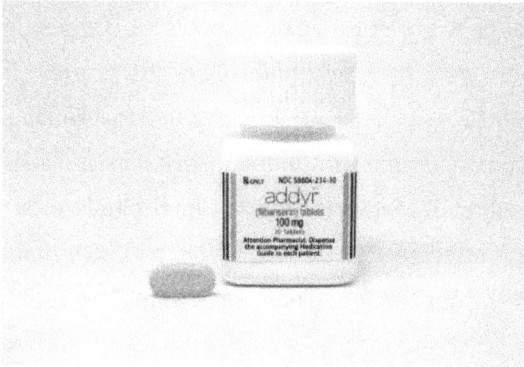

Figure: 36. Female Addy tablets

Fliban tablets were also discovered in America around 2009 for the treatment of loss of sexual desire in females. It is reported that Flibanserin was initially developed as an antidepressant for both men and women, but the drug was found to have little effect on people's mood. However, the majority of women who were enrolled in the clinical trials reported that the drug's side effect was that it makes women develop more interest in sex, besides drowsiness, dizziness and nausea.

The drug was then dropped in 2010 as an antidepressant, because of its limited effect and was soon being repurposed as a desire booster for women with hypoactive sexual desire disorder (HSDD). Further studies were conducted on the drug, which suggested that the drug does boost sexual desire although the effect is modest. One woman who was on the initial trial of Flibanserin in 2011, confessed that after a couple of weeks she was totally different person. She would wake up in the middle of the night and caress her husband.

Linda Geddes (2015) says more studies revealed that many women, who were on the drug, reported an increased number of satisfying sexual events. So today, female Viagra is used to treat young women and premenopausal women with acquired generalized hypoactive sexual desire disorder (HSDD) as characterized by low sexual desire that causes marked distress or interpersonal difficulty.

This medication is to be taken daily at bedtime. It appears that the medication can begin working within four weeks of treatment. How does the medication work? Scientifically, it has been found that Fliban targets the key neurotransmitters, or chemicals in the brain, that impact sexual response. The work of Fliban tablets is centred in the brain's prefrontal cortex. Here, flibanserin has a positive effect on chemicals in the brain involved with sexual excitement by increasing dopamine and norepinephrine. The medication increases the number of satisfying sexual events per month and can be used to treat female dysfunction, and is generally is sold under the trade name Addy. The side effects of the drug are dizziness, sleepiness, and nausea that can occur about three to four times or even more often.

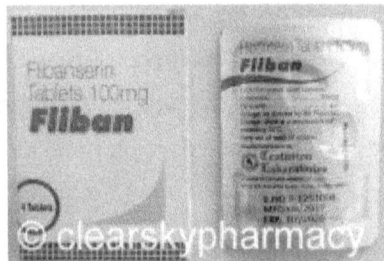

Figure: 37. Filban Tablets

However, when dealing with this medication, I want to reassure the readers that medical professionals have suggested that Flibanserin tablets should not be used for the treatment of low sexual desire caused by a medical or mental/mood disorder, problems in the relationship, or the effects of other medicines. In addition, this medication should not be used by women who have passed through menopause. Flibanserin tablets are not used to enhance sexual performance; this medicine is also known as female libido pills and sex increase tablets for women. Female Viagra can also be used to treat women with a condition called hypoactive sexual desire disorder, that is characterised by a lagging libido. It is reported that Serotonin receptor 1A and Serotonin receptor 2A antagonist can also be given to premenopausal women with low sex drive. If a woman does not want to take oral medication, she can receive counselling from a therapist who specialises in sexual and relationship issues by using a vaginal lubricant, if a woman is experiencing pain during sexual intercourse.

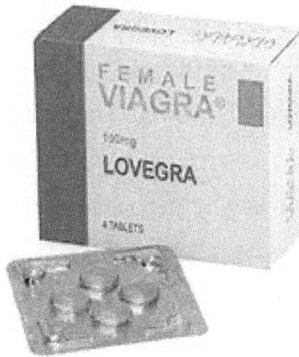

Figure: 38. Female Viagra

Keep in mind that sexual dysfunction is a problem only if it bothers you. If it doesn't bother you, there is no need for treatment.

What happens when a woman takes female Viagra? Since Viagra enhances sexual arousal in men by increasing the blood flow to the penis, female Viagra has a similar effect on women by increasing the blood flow to the female genitals and thereby producing better arousal sensation and lubrication in the genital area. It is taken daily at bedtime.

What is an orgasm?

An orgasm is a feeling of intense pleasure that happens during sexual intercourse (it is also called climaxing). In other words, an orgasm is the peak of sexual arousal when all the muscles that were tightened during sexual arousal relax. This is normally accompanied by the release of ejaculatory fluid (see figure: 28), and about 10 percent of women also ejaculate during an orgasm. Medical professionals and mental health professionals define orgasms differently. According to Newsletter: Medical News Today (2018), it defines orgasm as "The peak of sexual excitement. It is a powerful feeling of physical pleasure and sensation, which includes a discharge of accumulated erotic tension."

It appears not a great deal is known about the orgasm, and over the past century, theories about the orgasm and its nature have shifted dramatically. Healthcare experts have only recently come out with the idea of female and male orgasms in the 1970s, where they claimed that it is normal for both men and women not to experience orgasms. This argument tells us how scholars differ in ideology of orgasm. In my research, I respect the ideology of each scholar because he/she knows why they say so. However, what all the scholars have agreed on is that orgasms in both men and women are caused as a result of the continual stimulation of erogenous zones such as the genitals, anus, nipples and perineum.

What happens during an orgasm?

We do not know much about what happens during an orgasm, but I found that Masters and Johnson have attempted to explain this, and as such, we are going to use the four-phase model discovered by them to demonstrate about orgasm in human beings. Let us first examine male orgasm.

The male orgasm

Many people do not know that there is something important for a man touching a woman's inner thighs. By touching, feeling and kissing the inner thighs, this increases sexual thoughts and arousal in a man. When a woman is sexually aroused, she easily opens her thighs for a man to touch. This sends a signal of trust, and excitement in both. Both men and women benefit from physical closeness, and the immediate physiological rewards of oxytocin include increased immensity and lower stress. The emotional benefits are limitless.

Having said this, I would like to say that male orgasm can come through: -

▶ Excitement: When a man is stimulated physically or psychologically, he gets an erection. This is when the blood flows into the corpora (i.e. the spongy tissue running the length of the penis) causing the penis to grow in size and become rigid. At this time, the testicles are also drawn up toward the body as the scrotum tightens.

▶ Plateau: As the blood vessels in and around the penis fill with blood, the glands and testicles increase in size. In addition, thigh and buttock muscles tense, blood pressure rises, the pulse quickens, and the rate of breathing increases.

▶ Orgasm: Semen is made up of a mixture of sperm (5%) and fluid (95%). When a man has an orgasm the semen is forced into the urethra by a series of contractions in the pelvic floor muscles, prostate gland, seminal vesicles, and the vas deferens and is squirted out of the penis into the vagina — this is known as ejaculation. The average male orgasm lasts between 10-10 seconds. When a man has an orgasm, his heart may beat faster and his breathing may change. After this, a man would usually not have another orgasm for some hours or days. This is known as the recovery phase, when the penis and testicles shrink back to their normal size, and this can last from a few minutes to a few hours.

▶ Resolution: Soon after orgasm, a man enters a temporary recovery phase, where further orgasms are not possible. The length of the refractory period varies from man to man. This period lasts from a few minutes to a few days, when the man can go back to the point of sexual excitement. This period generally grows longer as the man ages, which means, and older man takes longer to get back to sexual excitement than a younger man, who can get back to sexual excitement in matter of minutes.

The female orgasm

A female orgasm is quite different to the male ones, and while it is known to last much longer, at the same time it can be a little tricky to reach the climax. Moreover, unlike men, most women need a little foreplay to reach their peak. There are certain pressure points which will help in making that journey to climax a lot smoother. In fact, according to a study conducted by the Journal of Sex and Marital Therapy, it found that 80% of women do not orgasm from penetrative sex. This means they cannot come to climax without clitoral stimulation (see figure 15 for clitoris). Therefore, this implies that if you want your woman to reach orgasm as expected, you need to put one of your fingers in and out of her vagina and explore her clitoris. Caressing and playing with it gently can help her reach a knee-jerking orgasm as the clitoris contains about 8,000 sensitive nerve endings. It is true that the clitoris usually becomes erect during sex, just like man's penis, making it highly erogenous. Breasts are also sensitive to sexual stimulation, so women can be turned on with proper touching or fondling. Some women can only achieve a climax through nipple stimulation. Therefore, it is up to the man to find out what works for his lady and continue accordingly.

Another point or area to sexually stimulate a woman is by softly touching her neck or back, because in these areas there are a lot of nerve endings. Having said this, I would like to say that female orgasm can come through:-

- ▶ Excitement: When a woman is stimulated physically or psychologically, the blood vessels within her genitals dilate and increased blood supply causes the vulva to swell, and fluid passes through the vaginal walls making the vulva swollen and wet. Internally, the top of the vagina expands. Like in men, the heart rate and breathing quickens and blood pressure increases.
- ▶ Plateau: As blood flows, the introitus (i.e. the lower area of vagina) becomes firm. Breasts can increase in size by as much as 25 percent and increased blood flow to the areola (i.e. the area surrounding the nipples) causes the nipples to appear less erect. During this, the clitoris pulls back against the pubic bone, seemingly disappearing.

- Orgasm: The genital muscles, including the uterus and introitus, experience rhythmic contractions around 0.8 seconds apart. The female orgasm typically last longer than the male at an average of around 13 — 51 seconds. Unlike men, most women do not a have recovery period, so they can have further orgasms if they are stimulated again. When a woman has a vaginal or clitoral orgasm, an intense pleasurable release of sexual tension is accompanied by contractions of the genital muscles. Some women may ejaculate when having a vaginal orgasm. A clear fluid spurts from glands close to the urethra during intense sexual excitement or during orgasm. These glands are called the Skene's glands. When a woman has a vaginal orgasm, she may be able to experience more than one orgasm shortly after the first if she continues to be stimulated.
- Resolution: Soon after reaching climax, the body of a woman gradually returns to its former state, with swelling reduction and the slowing of pulse and breathing.

Can a man increase the amount of semen he produces?

It is generally believed that a man can increase the amount of semen he produces by doing the following:

- If a man is a smoker, he should stop smoking because most smokers have lower quality sperm than non-smokers.
- If a man is having regular sex on a daily or weekly basis, he should avoid sex for some days or weeks.
- And if a man likes masturbation, he should stop it for few days. This would enable semen to be accumulated.
- Some men ejaculate very quickly during sex, so to increase the amount of semen, a man should delay ejaculation during sex.

Scientists have found that men are not the same when it comes to orgasms. Some of them can easily reach orgasm during sexual intercourse, while others don't reach orgasm during sex but rather they reach climax through masturbation, and yet others find it difficult to reach climax at all.

Difficulty in having an orgasm can be caused by several things, and the most common causes include:-

- ► Worries or lack of knowledge about sex
- ► Being unable to relax
- ► Not being stimulated or aroused enough
- ► Relationship problems
- ► Feeling depressed or stressed
- ► Previous traumatic sexual experience
- ► Erectile dysfunction (impotence)
- ► When testicles are not producing semen or producing just a small amount of semen (causing retrograde ejaculation)
- ► When a man has premature ejaculation, which means ejaculating too quickly
- ► When a man ejaculates too slowly or not at all (delayed ejaculation)
- ► Orgasm without ejaculating (anejaculation)

Some people think that an orgasm is an end in itself, but according to Pamela Supple, an expert in sex and relationship (2020), orgasms are as much a part of health as brushing your teeth or eating a healthy diet. She observes that orgasms play a huge role in women's overall health and wellbeing. William H. Masters and Virginia Johnson (1986) in their research about human sexual response, also found that sexual response such as excitement, plateau, orgasm and resolution in both men and women are not only limited to penile or vaginal intercourse. Although 1 in 3 women have trouble reaching orgasms when having sex, those who reach orgasms enjoy the effects an orgasm has on the body in different ways, as follows: -

- ► Orgasm helps with pain relief — the release of oxytocin is associated with pain relief.
- ► Orgasm leads to better sleep — it helps facilitate deep relaxation by boosting endorphin levels and flushing cortisol.
- ► Orgasm can regulate appetite — the hormones released during an

orgasm can energise women's hypothalamus gland, which helps women's body regulate appetite.

▶ Orgasm can keep one look younger — having regular orgasms can help slow down the ageing clock. They keep one looking younger for longer.

▶ Orgasm can improve digestion — there is general saying that climaxing provides and helps in the natural detoxification process in a body, which at the same time helps improve digestion and mood.

▶ A study published in 1997 suggested that the risk of mortality was considerably lower in men with a high frequency of orgasm than men with a low frequency of orgasm; this counter view is that the pleasure of orgasm is "secured at the cost of vigour and wellbeing".

▶ There is evidence that frequent ejaculation might reduce the risk of prostate cancer. A team of researchers found that the risk for prostate cancer was 20 percent lower in men who ejaculated at least 21 times a month compared with men who ejaculated just 4 — 7 times a month. Several hormones that are released during orgasm have been identified as oxytocin and DHEA. Some studies suggest that these hormones could have protective qualities against cancers and heart disease.

▶ Oxytocin and other endorphins released during male and female orgasms have also been found to work as relaxants.

Female orgasmic disorders

A study shows that female orgasmic disorders are always centred around the absence of significant delay of orgasm following enough stimulation. The absence of having orgasms is also referred to as "anorgasmia". Female orgasmic disorder can also occur as a result of physical causes such as gynaecological issues or the use of certain medications. It can even occur as a result of psychological causes of female orgasmic disorders such as anxiety and depression.

Many women have problems with sex at some stage in their life, known as female sexual dysfunction (FSD). Sexual problems affect around 1 in 3 young and middle-aged women, and around 1 in 2 older women.

Male orgasmic disorders

Male orgasmic disorders, like female orgasmic disorders, involve a persistent and recurrent delay or absence of orgasm following enough stimulation. It is very unfortunate that male orgasmic disorders could be a lifelong condition or one that is acquired after a period of regular sexual functioning. It also can occur as a result of other physical conditions, such as heart disease. Male orgasmic disorders in males can also occur as a result of psychological conditions, such as anxiety or through use of medications such as antidepressants. One form of sexual dysfunction that can adversely affect the quality of men's sex life is known as "premature ejaculation".

Premature ejaculation: Studies revealed that premature ejaculation (PE) is one of the common sexual complaints among men. This is when a man ejaculates within one minute of penetration of the penis into the vagina. It is a form of sexual dysfunction that can adversely affect the quality of a man's sex life. It can adversely affect sexual satisfaction for both men and women.

It is generally believed that premature ejaculation is likely to be caused by a combination of psychological factors such as guilt or anxiety, and biological factors such as hormone levels or nerve damage. In a majority of cases, an inability to control ejaculation is rarely due to a medical condition, although some doctors may not agree with this. As mentioned earlier, PE can lead to distress, embarrassment, anxiety and depression. One woman from Australia was telling her friend, "My husband always ejaculates as soon as his penis penetrates my vagina. I am not happy because I cannot reach orgasm as I expect to. For this reason, I want to look for a sugar daddy who can 'rock' my vagina." This is purely a distress and frustration that is common among women, who have husbands that have premature ejaculation.

A common drug used in many countries to treat primary and secondary PE is Dapoxetine, (the brand name is Priligy). This medication is used only if: -

► vaginal sex lasts for less than 2 minutes before ejaculation occurs.

► ejaculation persistently or recurrently happens after very little sexual stimulation and before, during, or shortly after initial penetration, and before he wishes to climax.

- there is marked personal distress or interpersonal difficulty because of the PE.
- there is poor control over ejaculation.
- most attempts at sexual intercourse in the past 6 months have involved premature ejaculation.

But remember when you are taking Dapoxetine that it has side effects which can include nausea, diarrhoea, dizziness, and headache.

Source: Newsletter, Medical Today, 2018, P. 3.

For Men

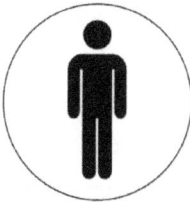

Get information about
problems with your erection,
premature ejaculation,
low sex drive and more

For Women

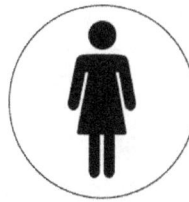

Answer your questions about
your low sex drive, and
difficulties with organism,
vaginal dryness and more"

For Couples

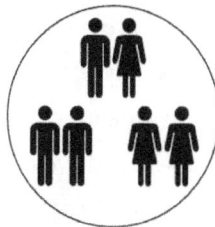

Learn about counselling options, sex therapy, how to
talk to your GP about sexual problems, and more.

Figure: 39. Sexual problems in men and women

Loss of Sex Drive: Loss of sex drive, also known as "libido", is when a person has a reduced interest in sexual activity or sexual thoughts. Losing sex drive is common among both men and women. It can be linked to many things such as relationship issues, stress, anxiety, some medical conditions and side effects of medication.

A reduced sex drive affects some women at certain times of life, such as during pregnancy, after having a baby, or during times of stress. But some women experience it at all time. The physical and psychological causes of libidos include:-

- relationship problems
- depression
- previous mental or physical trauma
- tiredness
- diabetes (both type one and type two diabetes)
- hormone disorder
- excessive alcohol consumption or drug use
- certain medicines, such as the SSRI type of antidepressants.

How does the Dapoxetine tablet work and how long does it last?

Dapoxetine/Priligy tablets increase the time it takes to ejaculate and can improve the control over the ejaculation. It starts to work very quickly; a tablet is taken when a man anticipates having sex, rather than taking it every day. A man must take it 1-3 hours before having sex. The drug is rapidly eliminated, and it can last approximately between 1-4 hours for the 30mg tablet.

Dapoxetine is a safe and effective treatment for premature ejaculation (PE). When taking Dapoxetine, a man should avoid alcohol, because alcohol can affect the effectiveness of the drug. The drug can be taken with Viagra or with Cialis. It must be used with caution, especially when a man is to take it at the same time as Viagra or Cialis.

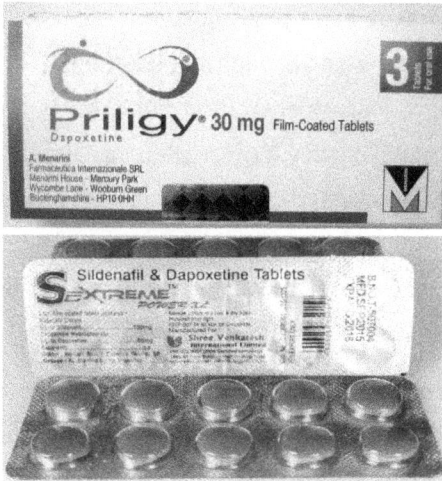

Figure: 40. Dapoxetine tablets

This drug cannot be purchased over the counter, so whenever you think you want to try it, please contact your medical doctor.

Summary of facts about orgasm

▸ Orgasms have multiple potential health benefits due to the hormones and other chemicals that are released by the body during orgasms.

▸ Orgasm do not only occur during sexual stimulation.

▸ People of all genders can experience orgasmic disorders.

▸ An estimated 1 in 3 men have experienced premature ejaculation.

▸ Trans people can orgasm after gender reassignment surgery.

▸ Orgasm does not have one universal definition.

Side effects of drugs use for male enhancement

Common side effects of Viagra:

We should not forget that every medication has its own side effects. Therefore, Viagra is not an exemption. The common side effects of Viagra include the following:

Firstly, it may make a penis larger but not hard. Secondly, it can make a penis hard but may not be hard enough for penetration. Thirdly, it could make a penis hard enough to allow penetration, but it may not be hard enough to complete the business. Fourthly, it can make penis completely hard and fully rigid. In general, Viagra makes the body of a man relax. In the vascular system, cGMP causes the walls of blood vessels to relax. It dilates the blood vessels, allowing blood to flow easily. Somewhat unexpectedly, this relaxation paves the way for an erection.

However, the most common side effects of Viagra can include headache, flushing, upset stomach, abnormal vision (blurred vision), stuffy or runny nose, back pain, muscle pain, nausea, dizziness and rash.

Harmful side effects of Viagra:

Coital Coronaries: Those who seek male enhancement after dealing with impotence may have other health issues. For instance, someone with coronary problems who has not had sex in some time should have a doctor check for serious conditions such as heart disease, diabetes and some types of cancer before taking Viagra. Using male enhancement drugs such as Viagra can prevent them from finding other problems and someone with cardiovascular disease can die suddenly during sex.

Side effects of Cialis:

According to John P. Cunha (2018) Cialis (Tadalafil) is a phosphodiesterase inhibitor used for treating impotence, which is commonly known as erectile dysfunction or ED). The most common side effects of Cialis include the following:-

- ▸ flushing (redness or warmth of the face, neck, or chest)
- ▸ headaches
- ▸ stomach upset
- ▸ diarrhoea
- ▸ flu-like symptoms like stuffy nose, sneezing or sore throat
- ▸ memory problems

- chest and muscle or back pain
- nausea
- low blood pressure
- dizziness
- blurred vision and changes in colour vision,
- abnormal ejaculation, and
- prolonged erections known as priapism.
- nose bleeding
- dry mouth
- increased blood pressure
- palpitations,
- increased heart rate
- fainting,
- stroke
- indigestion
- a painful or prolonged erection lasting 4 or more hours.
- sudden decreased vision (including permanent blindness, in one or both eyes
- a sudden decrease or loss of hearing, sometimes with ringing in the ears and dizziness.

This is not a complete list of side effects and others may occur. The recommended dose of Cialis is 5 — 20 mg per day taken before sexual activity. Cialis may interact with rifamycins, antibiotics, antifungals, antidepressants, and other drugs used to treat high blood pressure or a prostate disorder, heart or other medications.

How do you know if your partner is having an orgasm?

The majority of people around the world do not know when a partner is having an orgasm. Some of them take the cries of a woman in bed as having an orgasm, without understanding that this could be associated with pains or emotion.

However, Kendall (2011), in his article: *"How do you know if your partner is having an orgasm?"* observes that during an orgasm, hormones called endorphins are released into the bloodstream, causing intense pleasure and relaxation. People may feel flushed or warm and may experience rapid muscle spasms all throughout their bodies, but mainly concentrated in the genital and anal areas. Orgasm is the peak of sexual arousal when all the muscles that were tightened during sexual arousal relax.

A man's orgasm is usually accompanied by the release of ejaculatory fluid (see figure: 28), and about 10 percent of women also ejaculate during an orgasm. Women's experience with orgasm is more varied than men's, and not all women experience orgasm in the same way. It is often the case that a woman or a man won't have an orgasm during sex. That's perfectly normal. But some women are less likely to have orgasms than men.

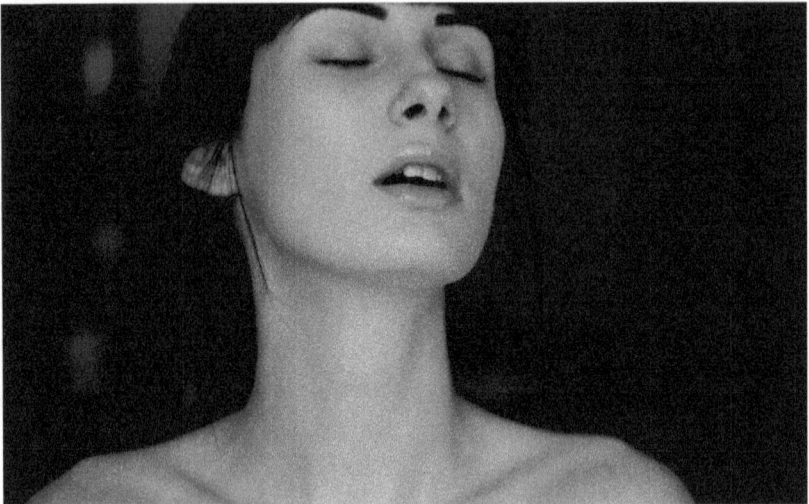

Figure: 41. Woman's Orgasm

With men, you can usually tell if they have an orgasm because they usually ejaculate. With women, it is not so simple because there is often no physical evidence. If you're concerned about knowing when and if your partner has an orgasm, talk about how you can let one another know before you have sex.

Letting partners know you care about making them feel good is a great way to show that their pleasure and enjoyment is important to you. (P. 4)

Chapter Ten
Dark and White Sides of Men and Women

The Origin of the term "Dark Side"

The term "dark side" is now becoming common among African Australians. However, not many of us understand the meaning and its origin. Generally, dark side means the evil and malevolent aspect of human personalities often referred to as "hidden" or "inner characters" of males and females. In other words, a dark side of a person is what people hate most in life such as fear of failure, extreme shyness or sexual compulsion; it is something to do with the selfish nature of a human being. Having said this, we should not be misled that the dark side is only found among the Africans. No, this is not true, it is found across Australian societies.

The phrase dark side originated from George Lucas in 1977, when he was producing his film, and he portrayed the dark side concept as the evil aspect of power control in the universe, which he called "force". This implies that the dark side of a person is the "negative" or "downside" of a person; and the "white side" of a person is the "positive side" of a person.

Here comes a question, "Is there dark and white side of a person?" The answer to this question is that nobody is perfect in this world and nobody is totally bad, in a true sense of the word. Therefore, every human being has both dark and white sides. Man has a good side, which is a tendency to show compassion and help others and a white side, that is a tendency to pursue dreams and interests at the expense of others.

The dark side usually breeds envy, jealousy, resentment, bitterness, anger, pride and fear to mention a few. The negative (dark) and positive (white) sides are all inherent in human beings that is why one of our primary goals in life is to develop the good side of us and make it dominant over the dark side. We must overcome or control our tendency to feel envy, jealousy, vengeance etc. This is what we call character growth.

More importantly, we should not let our good side completely overcome our dark side. Our dark side, although it is toxic to other people, can be rewarding to us. We need to be selfish sometimes. We don't have to avoid discomfort to live a meaningful and engaging life. In fact, a bit of anxiety or anger can propel us do great things.

In other words, do not strive to be an entirely "good person" or entirely "bad or evil person"; you should find the balance in your life. Therefore, if you are "too good", you will suffer a great deal, and if you are "too bad" that even makes you toxic to the human world.

It is good to know that dark and white sides are part of who we are, based on our upbringing and what we are exposed to on a daily basis. As we grow, everything around us influences us in some way or the other. For example, if you take a child and raise it in a blank room, with nothing but a bed and a toilet, and control everything he is exposed to, he will grow up reflecting whatever he was exposed to. It is a form of imprinting, like when baby ducks follow the first object they see, they imprint it as their mother. As we mentioned above, all of us have a dark side and it includes a quality we don't dare reveal to others. It is the traits we are ashamed of and embarrassed about. It is the traits others have rejected. It is the traits we believe deem us undeserving or unworthy of love.

As mentioned before, we are all human beings, and no human can be perfect. We make mistakes every day, every month and every year and some of us don't even realize our mistakes, subsequently this starts becoming our dark side.

Is our bad side hidden inside?

Yes, as we have discussed above, all of us have a bad side, but psychologists believed that this bad side is not really hidden in us; it is out there in the open for anyone to see, just like our good side. We are people with personalities and no matter what we do, we cannot hide it from the world.

Scientists say that our personalities have three-dimensional projections and people always perceive us only from the two-dimensional projections that they see from their prospective (which means they see subjectively and not objectively). Therefore, when the perspective is changed, the same projection of the same object would also change. It is understood that from the shapes and perspective class in Art class, the same object could appear different when observed from top view, bottom view, front and back views. The same applies to our personalities, they are complex shaped objects, and a human's brain has room for an infinite number of perspectives. The bottom line is that no two perspectives are the same. It's said that one man's meat is another man's poison. What one person likes about you, the other person would not like. If one thinks that he/she can hide their real self from the world, someone in a society will know and tell him/her that the bad side is someone's secretive nature, which is known first by the person but at the end of the day many people will know about it. Having examined the dark side of a person, I would like to conclude by saying that we cannot control what other people do or how they will respond to us in every situation.

We have just said above that the bad side is part of our life, what we are exposed to on a daily basis, and as such, no one should be troubled by it. One should rather focus on what one wants to do about it. The best way to improve is to talk about it to people you trust and try to understand their perspectives, and this can help you make your choices.

Having said this, I want to emphasize that the dark side of African Australians has contributed very much to the rate of divorce in the country that leads African communities to view single mums and single dads as bad people in the society. It is generally believed that children who grow up with both of their parents are eleven times more likely not to exhibit violent behaviour than children who grow up with just one parent. Furthermore, studies show that children who are raised by a single parent in Australia are more likely to have trouble in school than children who grow up with both parents. Finally, research suggests that children raised by a single mother or single father are more at risk for certain psychological and developmental problems.

With all this in mind, I want to say that separation and divorce among African Australians, is the key factor to the development of sugar relationships among them.

The biggest challenge in divorce and separation that the mother or the father may face is to make the children feel guilty for having fun with their other parent. This usually happens when some parents involve children in their marital disputes, instead of discussing the issues separately in the absence of children.

However, some African Australians think involvement in sugar relationships it is not as easy as they think — it is complex. Many of them take it for granted that once a person is involved in a sugar relationship, everything would be fine and right. This is not true; if someone decides to become a sugar daddy or a sugar baby, he/she should realise that there is a dark side and a white side to every person — which is also known as the *unknown character of a person*.

Thus, from my research, I have discovered that both men and women have their dark and white sides, regardless of where they come from or where they live. As a result, I thought it may be good to list down some of the common dark and white sides of men and women. Before I do this, I would like to make it abundantly clear that these dark and white sides are not only for the African Australians, but they are applicable to all men and women across the globe. I will start by listing the white positive sides of males and females. This will be followed by list of dark negative sides of men and women. In addition, I am also going to list positive and negative sides of single fathers and single mothers.

The white/positive sides of men

During my research, I have identified the "top 35 positive sides" of men and the information is based on information from 80 African informants and secondary information from different books I have read. These are not the only white/positive sides of men, as there are many more. They include: -

- ▶ Loving — giving affection to a woman as she deserves.
- ▶ Forgiveness — he is not vengeful, doesn't record present and past mistakes. Ready to forgive and forget.
- ▶ Loyalty — doesn't cheat or flirt with other women.
- ▶ Selflessness.
- ▶ Hard working.
- ▶ Thinks of others first.
- ▶ Has good communication — lets a partner know what he thinks and wants as nobody can read minds.
- ▶ Provider.
- ▶ Protector.
- ▶ Caring.
- ▶ Sharing loads.
- ▶ Gentle temper.
- ▶ Tolerance — when there are problems, can tolerate or endure suffering.
- ▶ Patience.
- ▶ Readiness.
- ▶ Reading of psyche.
- ▶ Always remains a soft speaker.
- ▶ Minimizes anger.
- ▶ Offers suggestions.
- ▶ Has a good job.
- ▶ Independence.
- ▶ Good leadership skills.
- ▶ Has a good knowledge of the things he wants.
- ▶ Truthfulness — being honest and transparent.

- Trust — has confidence in a partner.
- Appreciation — doesn't forget to thank for little things done for him or family.
- Persistence — never stops until he achieves his dream for a woman or family.
- Wisdom — can distinguish between right and wrong.
- Understanding — he understands others as well as himself. Understand his choices and decisions.
- Great in bed.
- Good listener.
- Supportive — is there when a woman needs help.
- Respect.
- Interested in a woman/partner.
- Believing.
- Self-control — has self-discipline to avoid gluttony, drunkenness, idleness and lust.

Dark or negative sides of men

- Unloving — not giving affection to a woman as she deserves.
- Unforgiving — he is vengeful and keeps records of the present and past mistakes. He is never ready to forgive and forget.
- Does not have loyalty — cheats and flirts with women unnecessarily.
- Selfish and thinks of himself first and thinks of others last.
- Lazy.
- Has bad communication — he doesn't care about a partner.
- Unable to provide or to help.
- Unable to protect.
- Does not care.
- Self-seeking and self-centred.
- Aggressive person.
- Intolerance — never endures suffering, gives up easily.

- Impatient.
- Unprepared for any support.
- Ignorant of psyche.
- Likes shouting at other people or boisterous.
- Gets angry often and easily.
- Lacks general knowledge and can hardly offer any suggestion.
- Unreliable.
- Depending on other people too much.
- Has bad or poor leadership skills and has no vision.
- Lack all necessary knowledge of the things he wants.
- A good liar — he is never honest and transparent.
- Untrustworthy — never trusts his own partner.
- Ungrateful — never thanks a person for a good job done for him or family.
- Undetermined — never reaches any decision on what to do for a woman or family.
- Lacks discernment — can't distinguish between right and wrong.
- Lacks understanding and common sense — he never understands himself as well as others. He hardly knows what to choose and which decisions to make.
- Performs badly in bed.
- He is a bad listener.
- Never support a woman — he is not there when a woman needs help.
- Disrespectful person.
- Disinterested in a woman/partner.
- Disbelieving of anything in human life.
- Lacks self-control — has no self-discipline, addicted to drink, idle and full of lustful thinking.

Positive/white sides of women

- Expresses love to a partner — gives affection a man deserves.

- Good communication — lets another person know what she thinks and wants. Nobody read minds.
- Supportive — Be more of a carer, praise and appreciate the man for achieving a milestone or overcoming fears.
- Has a heart that can accommodate men.
- Respect — respects a man as he is and not for what he has or does for her. Respects space. Everybody in marriage needs his or her own space. Respect in marriage is a must.
- Shows interest in a partner — not all that a man likes interests a woman. She must allow the man to pursue his interests. Learn about the things a man is interested in.
- Listen — Listening is crucial for effective communication. Therefore, listen and understand when your man is talking.
- Trust — have confidence in a partner.
- Honest — this is the basis for a trusting relationship. Relationships that last are based on honesty and truthfulness.
- Self-control — have self-discipline to avoid lust and being controlled by men.
- Have a degree of understanding.
- Loyalty — don't cheat or flirt with other men.
- Forgiveness — they are not vengeful, do not record present and past mistakes of a man. Ready to forgive and forget.
- They are appreciative — men need to be appreciated and praised. A good woman always tells her man how much she appreciates the little things he does for her.
- Pick the right fights — disagreement and differences sometimes can lead to fights. They are good at thinking and picking their fights wisely. They are persons who always think for themselves before picking a fight. They always ask, "Is it worth fighting for?"
- Have true selves — Women who are not comfortable with who they are, will not be comfortable revealing "their true selves" to partners.

- They are creative in bed — Men always want to hear that they are good in bed, to boost their confidence and make them feel like "the man". They are women who can tell their men after sexual intercourse, "You were killing me, but that is what I like!"
- Some women do not care about what husbands are doing with other women.

Dark or negative sides of women

- Does not give affection to a partner.
- Not good at communicating with her partner -She is self-centred, she does not want a partner to know what she thinks and wants.
- She never supports any person — she doesn't care whether a partner achieves a goal or not.
- She has a heart that hates men and cannot accommodate any man.
- Disrespectful lady — never respects a man as he is and what he does for her. Does not respect personal space. Doesn't care about marriage.
- Doesn't show interest in a partner.
- Doesn't listen to any man. Does not care or want to listen and understand when a man is talking.
- She is not trustworthy — she has no confidence in any man.
- Dishonest — does not tell the truth. She is good for nothing.
- She is an easy-going (loose) person; she lacks self-discipline and can hardly avoid lusting and selling sex to men.
- Has a low degree of understanding.
- Does not have loyalty — she cheats and flirts with other men.
- Unforgiving person — she is always vengeful and keeps records of the present and past mistakes. She never forgets any wrongdoing.
- Never appreciates nor praises any good thing done for her.
- Always looks for the wrong fights, never picks the right fights — disagreement and differences sometimes can lead to fights. They are never good at thinking and picking their fights wisely. They always

jump into the fights without asking whether it is worth fighting for or not.

► Are too pretentious — they are comfortable with who they are, and don't like revealing "their true selves" to partners.

► They are never creative in bed — they rarely enjoy sexual intercourse.

► They always want to know what their husbands are doing with other women.

Negative/dark sides of being a single father

► Worry every day.

► Develop emotional issues.

► Deceased income which may cause stress and result in poor health.

► Feelings of loneliness, stress and depression.

► Has a bad attitude of judging others based on his pre-formed opinions.

► May find it difficult to accept new relationships.

► Often overworks himself to sustain his life and the life of a sugar baby.

► Unable to discipline his children.

► Tempted to kill his ex, for causing him to lose his dowry and children.

► Spends too much money on a sugar baby rather than on his relatives.

Positive/white sides of a single father

► Has a soft heart that gives money and time whenever a sugar baby asks.

► Women like him and they are happy to forego their virginity as long as they get plenty of his money.

► He is always available for sex on demand.

► Has access to getting a new woman every 3 — 4 years.

Positive/white sides of being a single mother

A single mother always needs to balance her work life and personal life.

► Receive a monthly allowance from a sugar daddy.

► Freedom of movement and less responsibilities

- Being a single mother helps balance the needs of children.
- Is consistent with discipline — but most of the children get into trouble.
- Children under the administration of a single mother are resistant to facing challenges.
- Has more rights to get a new man and can leave the man at any time she wishes.
- Gossips more freely.
- Free to join groups of lesbians.
- Can demand more money from a sugar daddy to support her relatives overseas.
- Has more quality time to spend with kids.
- Being a single mother fosters a strong bond between mother and children.
- Being a sugar mother provides freedom to meet a sugar daddy anywhere and at any time (usually for sex).
- She has enough money for things she needs and wants.
- She is free to ask a sugar daddy to contribute for the cost of her new car.
- She is freer to choose whether to have more children.
- She is free to force her kids to deal with their own disappointments early in life.
- No more domestic violence — no more conflict resolutions.
- Personal financial freedom to a certain extent.
- Being a single mother provides an opportunity to develop a spirit of competition in parenting.
- Claims financial benefits from Centrelink, such as single mother payment, Income Support, Child Support and has better access to public housing.
- Access to government concessions for single mothers.
- Access to single mothers' network and social support agencies networks.
- Acquires and develops maturity as well as a strong sense of community.
- She has less mouths to feed (or cook for).

- More time for privacy.
- More secure and has more peace of mind.
- They are there for men to win love, especially for those who wouldn't get anyone.
- No more sharing of pain, tears, joy, tantrums and disappointment.
- There is no one to undermine her authority.
- Can decide to cook or not to cook.
- She can do what she wants and when she wants.
- Strong mother/child bonding — spending one-on-one time with children creates a unique bond.
- Strong sense of community — it takes a village to raise a child, many villagers will support the children including extended family members.
- Share responsibilities — children will understand their contributions to the complete family system.
- Maturity — when children see how hard their mother is working, this will force them to collaborate and work with the mother.

Dark/negative sides of being a single mother

- Has intimacy with a man for money and sex.
- She often feels extremely naïve and dumb.
- Enjoys the secret sugar relationships with men.
- Is disturbed when community members and relatives talk about her secret sugar relationships.
- She is stressed when her secrets are discovered.
- The new social life of being a sugar baby is distressful.
- Struggles to keep out of community gatherings for fear that her relationship with a man or men would be exposed.
- She is underprepared to be a single mother.
- She is too loose, having too much sex in order to promote her business.
- Too pretentious.
- Having aspirations for multiple men for sex, to earn money.

- Raising a child as a single mother is very stressful.
- Lack of access to child health services due to a shortage of funds; financially unstable.
- Lacks support in emotional battles.
- Difficulties in handling new decisions.
- Single mothers find it hard to maintain discipline in the home. (Being the only disciplinarian can give rise to the behavioural problems in children.)
- Feeling intensely sorry when her children envy their friends who live with both parents.
- Making a relationship with a man is somehow difficult when little children are jealous and suspicious.
- Not having enough time to look after children due to domestic work, paid jobs, and a sugar relationship; this often add to stress, fatigue and pressure.
- Decrease in income, which can affect how much time and money parents must spend for their children. Children may need to adjust to changes in time management.
- Financial issues may lead to poor health and secretive sex work. Single mothers work long hours to meet the financial needs of the family.
- Being a single mother may lead to mental health issues like stress and anxiety.
- Being a single mother can lead to self-neglect and frustration.
- Being a single mother reduces social connections and networking; feelings of loneliness, stress and depression.
- Fear of failure to raise children to meet their dreams and demands.
- Loss of self-esteem.
- Being abusive, aggressive and disempowered.
- Difficulty in adjusting to the new life.
- Difficulty in managing teen behaviour.
- Low parenting quality.

- Missing normal and romantic sex.
- Likely to lose children to "Child Protection" or children are more likely to leave home for unexplained reasons.
- A single mother has more trouble making ends meet and is less involved in her children's lives.
- Worries every day.
- Good at ordering a partner to do what she wants to be done.
- Is afraid to meet or talk to the wife of the man with whom she has a sugar relationship.
- Low parenting quality—long hours of working may make her miss her child's important school and other functions.

Conclusion

In conclusion, it is understood that on arrival in Australia, married Africans spend 3 — 5 years happily. As time passes by, they started to learn about assimilation policies into a multicultural society and more importantly, about gender equality. Experiences show that many of the African Australians did not understand what it meant by the words "gender equality". The African Australians redefined gender equality as *"Freedom to do whatever you want"*. But this is not a true definition of gender equality. Gender equality means the state in which access to rights or opportunities is unaffected by gender. In other words, we can say, *"gender equality is a belief that both men and women should receive equal treatment. People should not be discriminated against because of their gender"*. Let us go back to the definition of "gender equality" from the African Australians' prospective, is this what "freedom" really means in the Western World? Freedom is a noun, and it means the power or right to act, speak or think as one wants without interference. Generally, freedom mean a person has the right to do things that will not, in theory or in practice, be prevented by other forces. The best example of freedom can be found in a woman regaining her independence after a controlling marriage is over.

With those views in minds, African Australians prematurely began to abandon their rich, binding cultures. It is believed that some of Africans have done this because of ignorance, while others have done it because of the misinterpretation and misconception of freedom and gender equality, which has led to stress and depression.

Verbal reports revealed that misinterpretation of freedom and gender equality resulted in a high rate of divorce among the Africans living in Australia, which opened the door for single mothers and single fathers to do whatever they want. The single mothers and single fathers could not meet their material and sexual needs, therefore, this promoted sugar relationships. Some of them might have known stigma attached to such relationships, yet they decided to go ahead and continue secretly as we have seen in Chapters 3 and 4 -they changed the term "sugar daddy" to "brother or uncle" and "sugar baby" to "sister" to suit their purposes. However, at the end of the day it has become clear that all this was done so other people would not understand the hidden agenda about sugar relationships.

An African sugar daddy spends between $300 — $1,500 per month on a sugar baby. The men are doing this because they want women to keep their appointments. And for women, they are taking this money not just to keep the appointments but also to meet their daily rising demands. Subsequently, the research found that as women keep on with their sugar relationships, their "demands" have become more than the "supplies". However, this necessitates some women to become involved in multiple sugar relationships. Unlike the women, African men who are involved with multiple sugar babies, are more driven by their lust and pride of having sex with many females. It is very unfortunate that both men and women, who become sugar daddies and sugar babies, have failed to understand the consequences attached to sugar relationships — that is sexual transmitted diseases (STDs).

In my research, I have decided that it is not enough to just discuss or examine sugar relationships among African Australians, but it is also important to explore how a man's and woman's body functions, in regard to genital sores, menopause in women, thrush, and sexual dysfunction in men, because all these are connected to heathy sex.

Marriage or remarriage is part of human life, thus after divorce some single mothers, widows and single fathers want to remarry; this is perfectly heathy. Remarriage is teamwork; it requires both partners to put in their individual efforts to make things work. Just as a woman wants a good husband, the husband also wants a good wife.

Marriage has two purposes: the first one is *"growth in mutual love"* between the couple. This mutual love should open ways to a new life. The second purpose is *"education of the children"* both at home and in the school.

In humans, some of us think that sex is only for procreation but it is also for pleasure, connection, and increased emotional intimacy. Experiences show that when a woman reaches the stage of menopause, she struggles emotionally, her intimacy with people may be there but intimacy with her husband or sugar daddy may have gone. Study found that sex drive naturally declines with increasing age in both men and women.

Bibliography

Andrea Downey (2018), *Swollen in the Organs*, The Sun, UK

Aqmp.news.com.au (2019) -04/11/2019

Caroline Kee (2018), *13 Reasons why your vagina might hurt during Sex*, BuzzFeed. News *Female*

Cavalla Sandra and Warner, Lyndan (1999) *Widowhood in Medieval and Early Modern Europe*, Pearson Education Limited, Harlow, UK

Chibwinja Francis, (2005), BBC — *Why have a sugar daddy?*

Charles Carlton (1978) *The Widow's Tale, Male Myths and Reality in Sixteen and Seventeen Century England*, Albion, A Quarterly Journal concerned with British studies, Vol. 10, No 2, PP 118-129

Canberra Times, February 2018

Crossway (2013), The ESV, Gospel Transformation Bible: Grace for all of Life, Printed in the United States of America, Wheaton Illinois 60187, USA

David Huger (2018), *Marriage Problems: What Husbands Need to Know about Menopause.* www.focusonthefamily.com/marriage 20/12/2019

Dr Kyle Livie, (1019), A Cultural Historian and Associate Professor of History, Ohlone College

Dr Betty Dodson (2011), *Can all vaginas handle big penis?* www.dodsonandross. com 04/11/2019

Dr Nicola Gate (2019), *The Feel-good Guide to Menopause*, Harper Collins Publishers, Level 13, 201 Elizabeth Street, Sydney, NSW 2000, Australia

Dr Len Kliman (2020), *Polycystic Ovarian Syndrome, Symptoms, Signs of PCOS,*

Epworth Freemasons Hospital, Suite 101, 320 Victoria Parade, East Melbourne

Debra Rose Wilson, (2019), *Female Genital Sores* www.healthline.com 04/11/2019

Emma Johnson, (2019), *Who deserves to call themselves a single mom?* www.wealthysinglemommy.com.au 04/11/2019

Jeremy Nicholson, M.S.W. PhD, (2017), *10 Major Flirting techniques for women* www.psycholgytoday.com 20/09/2019

Jon Johnson (2019) *Myths and Facts about penis captivus* www.medicalnewstoday.com 04/11/2019

Jonnifewr Huizen (2019), *Everything you should know about Menopause: Let us talk about painful sex* www.healthline.com/health/menopause 19/12/2019

Gray Miller (2016)

Kendall (2011) In his article, *How do you know if your partner is having orgasm?*

Khan Ali (2016) *Why are older women more likely to flirt or attract men?*

Korin Miller (2019)*5 Ways your vagina can change after sex* www.glamour.com 20/09/2019

Marriage Missions International (2019) *Revolving and Reflecting the Heart of Christ within marriage* www.marriagemissions.com 11/10/2019

Merriam webster.com

Mia DeSoto (2018) *A content Analysis of sugar dating websites*, California State University, Sacramento, UAS

Michael J. Brien et al (2001) *Widows Waiting to Wed? Remarriage and Economic Incentives in Social security Widow Benefits*, University of Virginia, USA

Nancy Luke (2005) *Are Wealthy Sugar Daddies Spreading HIV?* Exploring Economic Status, Informal Exchange, and Sexual Risk in Kisumu, Kenya, Population Association of America, Los Angeles

Leone Muchano (2005), BBC-*Why have a sugar daddy?* 20/10/2019

Rebecca Ashkenazy-MD (2019), *What you need to know about Menopause*, Women's Health, USA

Senator Michel Forshaw (2011) Chapter 8, *Africans in Australia* www.aph.gov.au/parliamentacy/Africa 18/05/2019

Stephanie Watson and Tim Jewell (2019) *What Causes early Menopause?* www.healthline.com/health/menopause/causes-early 19/12/2019

Sugar et al (2015) *Student participation in sex industry, Higher Education responses and staff experiences and perceptions*, Journal of Higher Education Policy and Management, 37/4, 400-412

Susan Hart (2009) *Widowhood and Remarriage in Colonial Australia*, University of Western Australia, Australia.

Suzanne Falck (2018) *What Cause Genital Rash?* www.medicalnewstoday.com/arts 04/11/2019

Teresa A. Treat et al, (2016) *Men's perceptions of women's sexual interest: Effects of environmental context, sexual attitudes, and women's characteristics*, University of Iowa, Iowa City, IA USA

Tome Morrissey Swam (2017), *Tern Dating Tips for Widows and Widowers*, The Telegraph.co.uk

Traci C. Johnson, MD (2018) Menopause causes www.webmd.com/menopause causes 20/12/2019

William Kremer (2014), *Can Couples Really Get Stuck Together During Sex?* BBC News Magazine — UK.

Wright, LaNika L. 2019. *Negative Sexual Experiences and rape: understanding the relationship between adult and childhood sexual victimization and somatic complaints, psychological factors, and self-rated health in college women*, East Carolina University, USSA

www.ingramcontent.com/pod-product-compliance
Lightning Source LLC
Chambersburg PA
CBHW021900020426
42334CB00013B/410